CAPITATION
New Opportunities in Healthcare Delivery

CAPITATION
New Opportunities in Healthcare Delivery

David I. Samuels

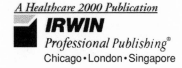
A Healthcare 2000 Publication
IRWIN
Professional Publishing®
Chicago • London • Singapore

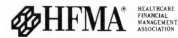
HEALTHCARE
FINANCIAL
MANAGEMENT
ASSOCIATION

A Healthcare 2000 Publication

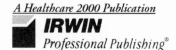

IRWIN
Professional Publishing®

This publication is designed to provide accurate and
authoritative information in regard to the subject matter
covered. It is sold with the understanding that neither the
author nor the publisher is engaged in rendering legal, accounting,
or other professional service. If legal advice or other expert
assistance is required, the services of a competent professional
person should be sought.

From a Declaration of Principles jointly adopted by a Committee
of the American Bar Association and a Committee of Publishers.

Irwin Professional Book Team

Publisher: *Wayne McGuirt*
Acquisitions editor: *Kris Rynne*
Marketing manager: *Cindy L. Ledwith*
Managing editor: *Kevin Thornton*
Project editor: *Carrie Sestak*
Production supervisor: *Pat Frederickson*
Assistant manager, desktop services: *Jon Christopher*
Jacket designer: *Palmer Design Associates*
Compositor: *Times Mirror Higher Education Group, Inc., Imaging Group*
Typeface: *11/13 Times*
Printer: *Buxton Skinner Printing Company*

Times Mirror
Higher Education Group

Library of Congress Cataloging–in–Publication Data

Samuels, David I.
    Capitation : new opportunities in healthcare delivery / David
I. Samuels.
       p.   cm.
    Includes index.
    ISBN 1–55738–640–4
    1. Managed care plans (Medical care)—United States.   2. Health
maintenance organizations—United States.   3. Medical care—United
States—Marketing.   4. Health facilities—Risk management—United
States.   I. Title.
    RA413.5.U5S25   1996
    362.1'0425—dc20   95–44282

Dedication

This book is dedicated to members of the general public, government, and general business communities who profess to know very little about capitated managed care, as well as to members of the provider community—most notably hospitals and specialty care physicians—who have so far seen little about capitation that they can truly respect.

Acknowledgments

Those who believe that writing a book is simply a test of individual willpower have probably never made it past the first chapter. To be sure, it took me six months to get past the first chapter, even with a detailed outline and two years of lectures and seminars on the subject firmly crystallized in my brain. Give me an audience, a microphone, and a time limit and I can deliver a top-notch presentation on what's wrong with capitated managed care and how the healthcare and non-healthcare industries can make it better. After the first 10 minutes, I can go into "automatic pilot" and say what I *need* to say in the given time. Talking about capitated managed care and my concepts of Reverse Gatekeeping®, Disease State Management®, and Capitated Enrollee Management is relatively easy.* Putting such thoughts into print is no longer an individual challenge.

My success at getting this important book written, designed, and published represents the successful collaboration of many people whom I am blessed to have known. This book would never have made it to print so quickly without the intuitive insight of Lisa Thomas Payne, who made the initial introduction of me to her friend at Probus Publishing. Let me digress on this initial contact, as my association at that time with Lisa was truly brief. People have asked me how one gets an entrée into the world of professional publishing, without first writing a manuscript and then paying an agent to sell it to publishing houses. I can respond only by saying that you have to find someone like Lisa on your own, which occurred as a combination of chance and plugging away within the speaker's circuit (she and I were presenters at the same seminar and read each other's materials; she later heard me speak and gave me an entrée to Probus on the spot). You never know when you are going to meet Lisa or me, or someone like us, but you can improve the odds that we will someday meet. To this end, you have to enjoy what you're doing until a good

---

*Disease State Management® and Reverse Gatekeeping® are registered trademarks of Comprehensive Care Corporation filed with the U.S. Patent and Trademark Office on July 12, 1995 and assigned serial numbers 74/702, 748 and 74/702, 749, respectively.

contact comes along. For me, the "plugging away" took two years. But finding the people in my life who have contributed to the coalescence of desires to get this book published has made the investment well worthwhile.

I remember giving Lisa's friend Kristine Rynne, acquisitions editor for Probus Publishing, a call, which involved a lengthy voice-mail pitch for two books. When Kris returned my call, we immediately connected, and Kris has since become one of my closest professional associates, even during the tense moments when I requested deadline extensions amid fears that someone named "Jimmy The Squirrel" would come around my house to break my kneecaps if I missed the next deadline. Or the next one. It was also Kris's genius that led to the design of the cover, one of the most compelling illustrations I've ever seen. In fact, it was the beauty and symbolism of the cover that helped motivate me to finish the last few chapters.

I owe a great thanks to the design staff at Probus, before the merger with Irwin Professional Publishing, who helped translate Kris's vision for the cover into an artistic reality. I am enraptured with the concept of the missing links in understanding capitated managed care, and the knowledge of them representing a ray of hope, opportunity, and prosperity in the creation of future capitated relationships, as well as in the retrofitting of Reverse Gatekeeping® within mature capitation markets like Southern California. This vision is what I see when I look at the cover of this book, and I'd like to acknowledge Kris, my pre-press editor Patrick Muller, and all of the other unsung heroes at Irwin Professional Publishing.

I appreciate the input from and validation of some of my research by my HFMA mentor Steven C. Holman, CPA, FHFMA. I also must thank my physician, Kenneth Kleinman, MD, for teaching me about the interrelationship of lifestyle and health status. I'd also like to acknowledge the personal encouragement given to me by my friend and associate Andrè van Niekerk, PhD; by my friend and mentor Norm Sigband, PhD; by my friend and colleague Jim Martinoff, MD, PhD; by my dear friend Patty Gardner, RN, MHA; by my friends Sean Lüus, MBA and Sylvia Merino, MBA; by my friend and breakfast buddy Fernando "Nando" Zepeda, MBA; and by my HFMA friends David Cohan, MHA, MBA, Catherine Klapper, MBA, CMPA, and Lawrence "Lan" Lievense, MBA, CMPA. All of the above individuals would invariably ask, whenever we'd have a chance to talk, "So how are you coming along on your book?" I can't say that I always answered them completely honestly when I said, "It's going great. I'm almost done." However, the word *almost* is truly a relative term.

The folks at Comprehensive Care Corporation, who came into my life during the last six months, must be thanked for believing in me enough to hire me and encourage me to achieve higher levels of accomplishment, this book being one of them. I am particularly appreciative of Drew Miller, CPA, MHA; Ronald Hersch, PhD; Chriss Street, MBA; Bernard Churchill, MD; and Michael Churchill, MBA. They have been especially supportive in helping me get the manuscript done and in allowing me to promote the book strongly.

Only a few people know how truly difficult it was for me to complete this book on a day in, day out basis. I'd like to thank my sons, Aaron Benjamin Samuels and Joshua Adam Samuels, for their patience and understanding, a true feat considering their ages of 12 and 9, respectively. While their friends (mostly male) were going on family vacations, getting quality time with their fathers, and having fun with their families, Aaron and Josh often (not always, of course) gave me the permission to "work on your book." The admiration they have of me, now that the book is finished and their names are somewhere in it, is priceless. Now they can point to something tangible as an example of the contribution Daddy made to the healthcare industry today and to their future. I hope everyone at some point in life makes a lasting contribution to society that merits the praise of his or her own and extended family.

I must also thank my parents, Melvin Samuels, MD, and Charlotte Samuels, MFT, for investing their love, respect, and trust in me for many years and hoping one day (someday) to see even a modest return on their investment. I'd also like to thank my *other* parents, Dorothy and Max Simons, for their love and encouragement during those troubling months when I kept rewriting Chapter One. I'd also like to thank my brothers, Mark, Joel, and Bruce; my sister-in-law Lisa; and my brother-in-law Joel I., for not discouraging me (yes, that is a compliment) even if they privately profess that they have no idea what I'm really saying. I hope that this book allows them to see inside my twisted brain and that I can repay the encouragement they've given me for so many years.

Most important, I must thank my wife, Lori. Lori was the one who took it upon herself to encourage me to write when I was confident that my writer's block was too crippling. Like the Annie Wilkes character in Stephen King's book *Misery,* Lori found many creative ways to encourage me to sit in front of the computer and write, most of them reflective of her love for me and her admiration of me (although if asked she'd deny it). Perhaps most encouraging was her obvious white lie (at least I hope it was) of, "You're never going to finish this book, because you never finish anything you start." Thank you, Lori, for believing in me and, in your own cryptic way, encouraging me to excel. I love you.

Finally, like everyone else, I must thank God. There is a reason for everything, even though we often don't come close to understanding everything. I hope this book helps others to understand more about capitated managed care and to recognize what many really don't understand. It is my hope that true understanding about *both* systems of capitated managed care comes to supplant the assumptions, misinformation, and basic confusion that often surrounds the subject. Thank you, dear reader, for keeping an open mind about capitation and for desiring to learn more, much more, about it.

Contents

Introduction

As a lecturer and educator from Southern California, I've seen the agonizingly clear light at the end of the tunnel when it comes to capitated managed care. Building a system based on capitation and subcapitation is a far cry from building a true health delivery system. One of the reasons I am writing this book is that my students sometimes say that their part of the country (say the midwestern or southeastern United States) needs such a system. Hence, one of the purposes of this book is to debunk the myths that Southern California has a system of "real" managed care and that Southern California should export what now passes for "managed care."

However, attempting to right wrongs or clarify the truth is not the main purpose of this book. I have trouble with the very term *managed care,* because it has become a trite expression that means many things to many people; furthermore, most payors and providers mismanage the managed care they have, and very little of what passes for healthcare is itself managed on anything other than a community level. After all, how can providers manage care they don't truly control or have the ability to predict?

The term *managed care* is frequently a misnomer when applied to preferred provider organizations (PPOs), which generally manage nothing but the pricing of contracts; the term is also misapplied to group- or panel-model health maintenance organizations (HMOs), often another misnomer. In order for care to be managed, providers need information about the inherent health of individuals. Not only is inherent health information needed for individuals but traditional principles of management are needed to call any care as being managed. Such management of care involves benchmarking against both the ideal state as well as the state of the beneficiary from the time of original assessment. In short, managing care should be no different from other forms of classical management: evaluating operational and financial data, maximizing the benefit of actions against their cost or their expected financial or operational return, gauging how efficiently resources are mobilized for expected returns, and so on. Classical management deals with controlling and changing known organizational structures and behaviors, improving the level of control for previously unknown or poorly known processes and organizations, motivating workers to provide maximum output from minimum inputs, and both controlling organizational costs and maximizing financial returns. The underlying necessities in such managerial processes are knowledge and the wisdom to use that knowledge appropriately.

In mature markets such as Southern California, the term *managed care* is a colloquialism for capitated managed care. Capitation is unrelated to the French form of capital punishment known as decapitation, although many healthcare providers would currently disagree with me. Since capitation exists as a provider risk-sharing vehicle transparent to consumers—with some subcapitation arrangements being transparent to payors—the public is rightly confused. Those who are aware of capitation see it as either a necessary evil or as symptomatic of the downfall of American healthcare. Without a retooling of capitated managed care to create or retrofit a health management system, such as my Reverse Gatekeeping® and Capitated Enrollee Management concepts, the "capitation-phobic" do have cause for concern.

Capitation itself is poorly defined in the healthcare industry. What is clearly defined, however, is the method by which capitation contracts are negotiated. This popular perception incorrectly assumes that capitation is a form of reimbursement on a pre-need basis. From this negotiation standpoint, capitation is simply the payment of a fixed sum of money based on a population of potential patients to one or more providers of healthcare services who assume the healthcare risk for such individuals for a period of time. The sum of money might be indexed in various ways to make it seem less fixed (e.g., adjusting for population-based demographics such as age, sex, and socioeconomic status). The provider accepting capitation might be a specialist or a primary care physician—or a coordinated organization of such physicians—who accepts less than total healthcare risk for a given population to make the enterprise seem less risky; of course, such physicians are paid less money for accepting less population risk. Regardless of the variations, however, the core contracting principle is still the same: Capitation involves providers who accept risk on a population basis and who are, it is hoped, armed with some appropriate information.

My good friend and colleague Dr. Andrè van Niekerk suggests that there is a hierarchy of information. At the basic level, there is a plethora of factoids in our world, some of them true and many of them false. The factoids may be spread by well-meaning friends and family members, gossip, an out-of-context encounter with a television talk show, or even respectable journals and newspapers. The factoids that are true and/or valid are reassembled into actual facts. An assortment of such facts that bear on one particular situation or event can become part of a body of data that can describe other or future events or occurrences, beyond the scope of previously collected facts. Different data, when analyzed in wildly divergent ways, can become sources of information. Similar patterns of information that describe divergent aspects of a single issue can represent a level of intelligence about a particular subject. Finally, years of evaluating intelligence can elevate the manager from the level of a spy or a master of counterintelligence; indeed, such managers possess unique wisdom unattainable at lower levels of information management.

As in the field of information management, the level of knowledge healthcare providers must have in order to manage care starts with the search for factoids. In the case of managed care, the search for factoids presumes that the manager requires a level of knowledge about the individual that is yet unknown. Yet the efficiency in collecting factoids depends on the ability of managers to engage in fact-finding. Just as a butterfly catcher needs binoculars, a net, and specimen jars, the fact-finding manager requires fact-finding tools: an open mind and the desire to find new facts; the means of searching out individuals with knowledge of factoids that, in the possession of learned individuals, could become new facts; some implement that can properly record factoids once they are encountered, ranging from a pad of paper and a pencil to a handheld, wireless personal digital assistant or subcompact computer; and, finally, knowledge of computerized database management and data modeling to retain factoids that have been captured, to create an environment where factoids can be processed into facts, and to reshape such factoids into wisdom-yielding intelligence.

This level of inquiry in the search for factoids is not yet occurring in the field of managed care, nor in most group- and panel-model health maintenance organizations. Most group- or panel-model HMO providers do not recognize that they lack the basic information they need to manage anything. This circumstance is indeed strange, in that the HMOs themselves are masters at collecting information and determining market and industry intelligence. That capitation even exists is a testimony to the intelligence-gathering and fact-management skills of HMOs, the darlings of the health insurance industry.

Finally, I feel I should mention that rationally managed systems that utilize capitation as a payment source have broader implications for future healthcare reform. In addition, properly functioning capitation-based systems can afford the creation of multinational approaches to improving health status and health management around the world. This potential can be effected by the use of some of the emerging technologies such as the asynchronous transfer mode (which facilitates the bidirectional transmission of huge databases as well as presentation-quality video images); advances in fiber-optic networking, cellular and satellite uplinks/downlinks, electronic medical records, and centralized data repositories; and eventual compilations of statistically reliable ambulatory outcomes data.

I have a dream that a truly managed health delivery system can rationally utilize capitation as a risk-assumption/compensation vehicle without shortchanging the public's need to become healthier and more health-focused consumers while preserving the providers' needs for critical information, improved provider–client relationships (1990s style), improved public health status, and an approach that de-emphasizes market share and competitive threats (even from nonphysicians), as well as—and perhaps most important—the opportunity for financial profit. Capitation can be a vehicle for providers to have better, more meaningful, and longer-term relationships with their vendors; for poorly funded public health systems to become attractive to private-sector providers using the Disease State Management® and Reverse Gatekeeping® techniques explained herein; for the marketplace to demand and accept a wider variety of capitated providers, whether providing traditional Western-based medicine or less traditional whole-body care; and for non-healthcare vendors around the world (who depend on the U.S. healthcare delivery system for substantial income) to redesign their pricing and products for a capitated marketplace, including exploring their own capacities for bearing risk. In short, capitated managed care can transform itself from a self-limiting payor classification for the healthcare industry to a new opportunity for healthcare delivery in the twenty-first century.

Chapter One

The Importance of Capitated Managed Care

Healthcare providers who think managed care will go away are sadly mistaken. True, the term *managed care* has been overused, and most providers assume that managed care is just about managing costs. However, managed care, especially *capitated* managed care, means a whole lot more, considering that the healthcare industry has been dealing with managing costs since the enactment of Medicare some 30 years ago. Businesses dependent on the U.S. healthcare industry (whether representing providers or nonproviders, whether domestic or international) need to learn about capitated managed care (1) because the U.S. healthcare delivery system is moving in this direction, (2) because capitated managed care will become the predominant payor source by the year 2000, and (3) because understanding and positioning for a capitated managed care marketplace will determine the ability of healthcare providers and non-healthcare enterprises dependent on this industry to remain in business in the next decade, and the extent to which they will do so.

We in the healthcare business have never really tried to make non-healthcare enterprises understand our industry, but I feel the transformation of our business to capitation should be changing this old perspective. Our perspectives of the world around us—that is, our *paradigms*—need to change just as our industry is changing. The perspective of non-healthcare enterprises should facilitate this transformation. For example, a telecommunications business might find that some 60 percent of its bottom-line income is derived from healthcare–oriented consumers such as physicians, general acute care hospitals, behavioral health hospitals, long-term care facilities, life care facilities, specialty hospitals, clinics, home health agencies, healthcare billing- and collection-oriented agencies, health maintenance organizations, healthcare payor organizations (including health-oriented insurance companies), and such evolving

1

entities as managed care organizations and accountable health plans. From a telecommunications standpoint, these healthcare enterprises might be using traditional equipment (such as telephones, regular business telephone lines, WATS lines, and PBX equipment); nontraditional equipment (such as fax, paging, cellular, and fiber-optic equipment; local and wide area network and gateway equipment and cabling; ISDN boards, software, and access fees; and telemedicine-oriented equipment, software, and transmission protocols, all operating over an increasingly fiber-optic network); and new products being targeted for this industry (such as telephony; satellite-based communications; cable-TV-based health information; electronic medical records with offline storage and instantaneous retrieval; and access to an ever-growing, and increasingly statistically valid, central data repository).

As they move into more capitated forms of revenue generation, these healthcare customers will increasingly develop budgeting and expense-management infrastructures that are tied to increasingly capitated incomes. When these infrastructures change, vendors (such as telecommunication enterprises and any other businesses that must continue to sell to increasingly capitated healthcare enterprises) will be under severe pressure to assume increasingly greater risk and sell on an increasingly capitated basis. If such businesses do not understand this trend, do not understand the basics of capitation, and do not comprehend the tremendous opportunities under capitation, they will jeopardize increasingly greater sales to the U.S. healthcare industry. This loss of income, especially for many firms that are 50 percent or more dependent on the U.S. healthcare industry for their own sales, will bankrupt those companies that don't improve their knowledge of capitated managed care and change their paradigm—and quickly.

THE NEW PARADIGM

A *paradigm* is a specific approach to a particular issue; it's how we come to understand something new or something old that we consider in a new light. True managed care represents a change to payment structures that does not require care management paradigms to change accordingly. Because of the scary nature of change in our society, particularly within the healthcare industry, our care management paradigms did not change significantly enough when previous payment structures changed.

Example: DRGs' Effect on Providers' Adopting "The New Paradigm"

Different approaches to managing care have been in the literature for many years, but very few concern how managing care changes when payment structures radically change. In 1983, when the U.S. Health Care Financing Administration (HCFA) changed the Medicare program to one of prospective payment, three very significant changes occurred. The first change, which the healthcare industry noticed the most, was the creation of over 400 diagnostic related groups (DRGs), which created rather fixed pricing for acuity-adjusted, inpatient admissions. The healthcare industry mobilized rather quickly to maximize its DRG reimbursements, primarily by reorganizing medical records and billing departments, purchasing coding systems and decision-support equipment and software from a burgeoning healthcare information systems industry, and educating healthcare providers to fine-tune their diagnoses and billable procedures, preferably in ways that maximized DRG reimbursements. The industry also began a process of "cost shifting," whereby increasingly greater portions of inpatient operations could be excluded from DRG rates and the charging structures could be shifted to less-fixed, and increasingly greater offsetting, levels. In short, the healthcare industry adapted its status quo to minimize the effects that DRGs would have on traditional income levels and overall operations (with medical records and the business office becoming minor casualties of change).

The second major change that occurred with the shift to prospective payment was the policy reversal of Medicare's previous encouragement of increased healthcare costs. Some healthcare businesses have responded to this change, but much less abruptly than to the rapid change in billing- and coding-oriented infrastructures since 1983. Prior to DRGs, Medicare reimbursed hospitals on the basis of their stated costs plus a 10 percent profit factor. We know from history that for-profit hospital chains (like HCA [now Columbia/HCA], Humana, and NME/AMI [now Tenet Health Care]) did not exist prior to the enactment of Medicare in 1965. These companies quickly learned that our government would reward their expansion, particularly if they could acquire hospitals and build increasingly specialized infrastructures, following which they would revalue their assets, submit new (higher) cost reports to the Health Care Financing Administration (HCFA) for providing care to Medicare beneficiaries, and receive 10 percent higher reimbursement levels over increasingly greater cost bases. To make matters worse, the government used to advance hospitals the money (from yet-to-be-filed cost reports) in the form of periodic interim payments (PIPs), which inevitably burned holes in their pockets. Hospitals created new levels of infrastructure, particularly in caring for Medicare patients, such as respiratory therapy departments (a function, prior to the enactment of Medicare, performed by registered nurses, who are still trained in nursing schools to intubate patients in respiratory distress); since the enactment of Medicare, we've created entire departments and job classifications to perform respiratory treatment at overall higher cost. At the same time, the industry saw meteoric growth in emerging industries such as diagnostic radiology, therapeutic radiology, computerized tomography, physiological monitoring equipment, ultrasonography, and cardiac-related imaging and testing, all of which were ready to accept PIP money from hospitals. The point here is that DRGs represented relatively fixed pricing. Respiratory therapy, since it's performed primarily for Medicare inpatients, becomes a cost under DRGs instead of a revenue source, yet very few hospitals have eliminated their respiratory therapy departments and redirected RNs (with applicably higher compensation) to intubate and add respiratory therapy–related services to their duty lists. In another example, central supply and central sterile supply—which, prior to DRGs, represented the lion's share of a hospital's revenues—became cost centers under DRGs, yet hospitals are still slow in responding to this rather major change; continuing to buy more disposable central sterile supply items, usually at tremendously higher costs, rather than even considering previously used, multiuse items that could be sterilized rather inexpensively in autoclaves or increasing their use of reusable uniforms as opposed to much higher-cost disposable ones.

The third major change was the creation of the prospective payment system itself. A prospective payment system is no longer a retrospective (i.e., reimbursement-based) payment system. Adopting a prospective payment system orientation is part of "The New Paradigm." In what should have been a very substantial effort by the healthcare industry to reorient its financial, operational, and overall budgetary infrastructures to an increasingly capitated basis of Medicare income, the industry has chosen not to respond and instead to treat DRGs as a new form of reimbursement. In so doing, the healthcare industry remains out of step with further refinements and changes to an increasingly widespread prospective payment system that continue to occur and extend well beyond Medicare to other third-party payors (such as insurance companies, health plans, Civilian Health and Medical Program for the Uniformed Services [CHAMPUS], and Medicaid) and even cash-based business (such as from other providers). The healthcare industry is starting to pay the price for not embracing "The New Paradigm," especially as providers try to force-fit capitation paradigms into a reimbursement structure that is as ill-fitting now as it was when DRGs first changed the industry.

The New Paradigm and the Move to Capitation

With the creation of the prospective payment system, HCFA gave hospitals fair warning that Medicare was no longer a form of reimbursement but rather an interim step toward a uniformly fixed method of pricing, paid in advance, that was increasingly less tied to actual hospital expenditures or care consumption. The ultimate extension of this form of payment, whereby all revenues are fixed, are paid prospectively, and are not tied at all to care consumption is known as *capitation* (see below).

The creation of a prospective payment system by HCFA, which included DRGs as a basis of payment in 1983, was the change most ignored by the healthcare industry and the one with the gravest consequences for capitated managed care. The ignoring of the creation of a prospective payment system has clouded the objectivity of the healthcare industry in other ways: While money has been spent to retool billing, coding, and charging systems within hospitals, little has been spent (or is even spent today) on improving access to clinical data that would allow providers to understand the true health status of their patients, to create information-based processes to help their patients stay out of the hospital (reduce consumption), to improve the value that patients and society derive from healthcare providers (outcomes), and eventually to enable people, especially those with chronic medical conditions, to take responsibility for their own health status (true health maintenance and eventual wellness management). These forms of data are part of the new paradigm for what providers need to know in an increasingly capitated world, but they typify what providers don't know they need or even could have. The data don't have to be created from scratch; in fact, much of these data exist today in the bowels of providers' computer systems—and in many vendors' computer systems as well—but are either thrown away or are otherwise inaccessible for modeling applications.

Capitated managed care represents a substantial extension of the managed care paradigm, for which old constructs and old responses (including those mobilized to deal with the evolving managed care paradigm) fall noticeably short, and are generally inapplicable. Clearly, with no change needed to care management systems imposed by the financial changes under the managed care paradigm, providers could treat managed care as a financial hoop through which they have to jump to get paid. For example, charges incurred for hospitalization under a managed care plan can be denied if there were no preauthorization for the admission; after a few such denials, hospitals that hire case managers can make sure that all of a health plan's required procedures are followed so as to prevent denials of charges. Furthermore, some hospitals are taking the extraordinary step of having case managers contact patients during preadmission to ensure that every admission is preauthorized.

Case management is also an example of the shortcomings of the healthcare industry's current attention: The emphasis is on obtaining the preauthorizations in order to submit claims for reimbursement and on reducing the lengths of stay, particularly for patients for whom "reimbursement" is sought from capitated payors. The industry's attention is not directed to understanding the consumption behavior under capitation of providers and their patients, so as to understand the determinants of unreimbursed consumption and potentially reduce demands for future healthcare consumption (also unreimbursed). Case managers could have been doing outcomes studies since 1989, which might have yielded a statistically valid, predictive model of appropriate healthcare consumption available today. Instead, hospitals ignored outcomes studies until about 1994—when the Joint Commission on Accreditation of Healthcare Organizations (JCAHO) first started requiring such studies as a condition of accreditation—and ignored the capability of case managers to perform them. Today, case managers are hired most often for their abilities to obtain preauthorizations and to impact lengths of stay, and less often for their statistical and data-modeling abilities. In fact, to this day, many hospitals continue their tunnel-vision orientation by collecting and maintaining clinical severity adjustment, patient satisfaction, and patient outcomes data (whether done by clinical staff—such as case managers or utilization managers—or by nonclinical, administrative staff) only because JCAHO mandates that they do so, but they utilize none of the data to improve clinical processes, change provider behavior, change caregiver attitudes, and/or improve patient outcomes data.

THE OLD PARADIGM

The protection of the status quo, what I call the *old paradigm,* is a powerful self-interest in this country. For example, the American Medical Association was vehemently opposed to legislative efforts of Congress to enact Medicare and Medicaid back in 1964 and supported an alternative "Eldercare" bill, which would have placed the responsibility for caring for seniors on overburdened state governments. Even then the fear was that "socialized medicine" was an evil American society could not endure. Yet what is it about medicine that could have socialistic implications?

The ill-fated Eldercare bill had some socialistic overtones as well, in that it would have enabled older Americans to receive disproportionately more public services than younger and middle-aged Americans; in most all states, a means test was applied to potential beneficiaries so that only older Americans most in need of public funds would be entitled to the benefit. Politically, the bill would have replaced then-current entitlements to Old Age Survivor's benefits, and would have coexisted with entitlements to the blind and the disabled—all of which were administered by the states. It should be also be noted that some states had more funds available than others for these limited entitlements and that the dollar amount of such benefits differed from state to state. Not only would there have continued to be polarization between the "haves" and the "have-nots," but the system further differentiated among the haves according to their state of residence, thus increasing the potential for "spillovers" to those states with the best monetary benefits, that is, the migration of specific populations from poorer states to adjoining richer states for better benefits.

Why "The Old Paradigm" Needs to Be Changed

A series of entitlements under any system that polarizes the American population into haves and have-nots is socialistic, regardless of the level of commitment to our hallowed free-market economy. The passage of Medicare and Medicaid, in my opinion, had more socialistic implications than many physicians would have then realized. A move by the 1995 Congress to reintroduce means testing for Medicare coverage appears to breathe new life into the AMA's Eldercare proposal from 1964.

In this country, and to this point in time, health or healthcare (there is a difference!) is not a universal right for all Americans. However, the enactment of Medicare ensures that healthcare is a right for the following classes of people:

• *Elderly*—Americans at least 65 years of age, regardless of income status, have a right to healthcare.

• *Blind*—Americans who are legally blind, regardless of income status, have a right to healthcare.

• *Disabled*—Americans who pass federal criteria for being "totally disabled," regardless of income status, have a right to healthcare.

• *Emergent*—Anybody living in the United States is entitled to a triage assessment of an emergent condition in a hospital emergency department (an assessment that typically lasts only a few seconds) under the "antidumping" statutes of Medicare, including those people ineligible for the Medicare program. In this manner, Medicare is also a means of assuring that everybody living in the United States has a de facto right to some form of assessment of a condition that could constitute an immediate life threat. However, care beyond that initial assessment is only a right for those (regardless of other entitlements) who would imminently die without any interventional care. In this case, the level of care anybody is *entitled* to receive is limited to that which results in the stabilization of the original condition or in unpreventable death. The only other limitation to this inalienable right to limited, emergency healthcare is to those who are known to have durable powers of attorney for healthcare (DPAHC) or other known "standing orders" waiving their rights to resuscitative care or conversional intervention. Such orders would have to be taped to the patients' bodies, in plain view, to ensure their being followed in the case of an accident or an unforeseen trauma that results in their being brought to an emergency department. With the exception of DPAHC, the voluntary cessation of life is still a crime in most every state.

• *Indigent*—Under Medicaid, healthcare is also a right for those who meet one of several income limitations to be classified as "indigent." Some counties also extend healthcare coverage to indigent individuals who might not qualify for Medicaid (such as homeless individuals who might not be able to supply an address required for Medicaid coverage). Depending on the state, such entitlements could apply to individuals who are not inherently indigent (for example, if the definition requires that household income fall below the poverty line established by the

U.S. Bureau of Labor Statistics) but would become indigent when the costs of medical care are taken into account along with other allowable household costs.

• *Detainees*—Healthcare is also a right for those who are incarcerated or involuntarily detained, regardless of American citizenship. Such healthcare could apply to most all detainees: to both convicts and unconvicted individuals awaiting trial within a detentional facility, to aliens awaiting deportation in a detentional facility of the U.S. Immigration and Naturalization Service, and to at-risk psychiatric patients involuntarily committed to a licensed facility for an initial 72-hour stay.

• *Neonates*—Finally, welfare and Medicaid (and therefore healthcare) are rightful entitlements for poor infants of another country born in the United States, who become virtually automatic American citizens. (Through our current immigration laws, non-American parents of an American neonate—either a naturalized citizen or an alien born in the United States who is entitled to receive public benefits—can fairly easily become U.S. citizens as well, and can also receive public welfare and healthcare benefits.) This perk is one of the chief reasons that poor, third-trimester pregnant women of other countries are attracted to U.S. hospitals for maternity care, typically accessed through the emergency department.

That these populations are entitled to healthcare while the populations that support them are not creates divisiveness and enmity. The effect is to polarize populations between the haves and the have-nots. For example, some members of the middle class not covered by managed care plans are covered by "major medical" plans, which, because of deductibles, do not entitle them to physical exams, whereas public healthcare programs for detainees, incarcerated criminals, and the indigent pay for such exams, as well as for less major healthcare needs. This polarized system is wholly unfair, unjust, and inherently wrong.

A new paradigm is needed for healthcare in this country, starting with entitlements but most important to ensure accessibility to care that is balanced between quality and price and not just price alone. This lack of balance is the real crime of panel- and group-model managed care plans, particularly under what passes for capitated managed care today, that make price-determined care an example of rationing.

In his book *Not What the Doctor Ordered: Reinventing Medical Care in America,* (Chicago: Probus, 1994) Jeffrey C. Bauer notes that the medical establishment represents an all-encompassing provider that participates in monopolistic behavior to the exclusion of nonphysicians (who, in specific cases, have superior or valuable, complementary knowledge that physicians generally do not possess). Consider the following examples, based upon Baver's work, which indicate the fallout of managed care under a framework that perpetuates price rationing:

- Why should non-trauma emergency care under capitation be rendered by board-certified emergency physicians operating in a hospital emergency department and not by family practice residents operating in an urgent care center?

- Why should a healthy woman's baby (free of complicating prenatal conditions) be delivered by an obstetrician (typically via C-section) operating in a hospital and not by a certified nurse midwife (or even a lay midwife) operating at home or in a freestanding birthing center?

- Why does stroke (cerebrovascular accident) care need to be rendered by a physiatrist in a rehabilitation hospital accredited by the Commission on Accreditation of Rehabilitation Facilities (CARF) or JCAHO and not by a general practitioner operating in a non-CARF-accredited or a non-JCAHO-accredited skilled nursing facility?

The only legitimate way to justify the added expenses that typify the status quo of the current healthcare delivery system is to show "value added" in higher-cost services compared with lower-cost ones. If the payor refuses to consider the value added and remains resolute on paying by price alone, the provider is stuck with either making do with the cheapest levels of care, subsidizing the costs of the higher levels of care, or devising alternative scenarios that may improve quality at increasingly acceptable levels of cost or may represent more acceptable tradeoffs in quality and price.

Providers manage best when they call the shots rather than depending on nonclinicians to call the shots. The best solution of all is to assume risk. The best vehicle for assuming managed care risk is capitation.

THE NEED FOR CHANGE AND NEW PARADIGMS

There is something to be said for how providers handle change. If providers are so enamored with maintaining the status quo at the expense of properly positioning themselves for formative change, they will almost certainly miss a valuable opportunity. Much can be said about the role of physicians' professional associations in supporting the transition of our healthcare industry to managed care. As late as November 1994, the American Medical Association took a position against capitated managed care, by arguing that the system itself creates rationing and undermines efforts of the association to improve quality of care and overall health status. This book will show that *there is no system for capitated managed care* and that *rationing is a logical response for having to manage without needed information.*

To most every provider, payor, and consultant I have found, capitation is viewed as merely a new compensation strategy for providers, a new form of reimbursement, even though such a view should have died with the creation of Medicare's prospective payment system through the introduction of DRGs. To be sure, providers consider capitation to be virtually unrelated to the provision of care and to current efforts to reduce utilization and improve overall quality of care. Furthermore, the classic definition of capitation could lead to this conclusion.

Capitation Defined

The classic definition of *capitation* is the following: *A method of payment for healthcare services in which the provider accepts a fixed amount of payment per subscriber, per period of time (typically in monthly increments) in return for providing all specified services over a specified time period.* As discussed in Chapter Four, this definition has many drawbacks, especially as they relate to operational wisdom that providers can readily use.

The Status Quo versus New Paradigms for Managed Care

The new paradigm represents changing care management according to changes in financial management inherent in capitated managed care. In its most simple state, the reality of this paradigm is this: If providers lose money when care is consumed, systems for managing care must change to reduce individuals' reliance on consuming services. The status quo paradigm itself represents a reliance on consuming services. The systems and resources are not mobilized for individuals until they become patients (e.g., they are scheduled for surgery, they are scheduled for admission, or they enter the emergency department). From this point, the case manager springs to action, the business office creates a patient and/or guarantor financial account, the medical records department creates a chart number, and a discrete record is created in the computer system.

But these systems spring to life only when a person is scheduled to, or actually does, consume services. If the financial realities of capitated managed care dun a provider when services are consumed, then why do systems within the status quo paradigm require consumption of services? Surely, the mobilization of case managers and decision support systems will reduce the amount of money providers will lose under capitated managed care; hence, the status quo paradigm exists under capitated managed care as a strategy to lose money—albeit less money. Why is the healthcare industry so willing to hang on to this money-losing strategy when previous money-losing strategies in our history were very quickly abandoned? Why is the healthcare industry so enamored with this money-losing strategy and so reluctant to adopt the new paradigm for managing care under capitation—a definite money-making strategy?

One rationale is that the need for a new paradigm is not easily apparent, as long as the status quo paradigm accepts managed care as a procedural hoop. Relegating managed care to a series of hoops is proving to be a shortsighted strategy. When providers consider managed care as a series of hoops, there is no real change in the paradigm of managing care: There is no change in the *way* care is managed, just in how well the status quo system of providing care is compensated—for better or worse. Yet the original question about our industry's fascination with preserving the status quo to its own detriment is still valid.

THE REALITY OF MANAGED CARE

That managed care is just a new series of procedural hoops or a new compensation practice is a troubling myth. Anyone who believes in this myth does not understand the reality of managed care. In practice, managed care is an all-encompassing paradigm, including everything from an attempt to manage healthcare consumption—such as utilization review and case management—all the way to capitation and other population-based pricing mechanisms. The statistics on the pervasiveness of managed care are also confusing, in that they show a substantial increase in managed care as a payor classification but don't distinguish how the term is being defined.

For purposes of this book, *managed care* is defined as *a means of providing healthcare services within a defined network of healthcare providers who are given the responsibility to manage and provide high-quality, cost-effective healthcare.* Curiously, the term is increasingly being used to include preferred provider organizations (PPOs) and their hybrid organizations—such as exclusive provider organizations (EPOs) and accountable health plans (AHPs)—and even forms of indemnity insurance coverage that incorporate preadmission certification and other utilization controls (see Chapter Two).

From my research, I have found that the term *responsibility* is the critical element that is increasingly defining what is and is not managed care and is planting the seeds of the paradigm shift itself. In managed care frameworks that include PPOs (and hybrids) and other utilization-managed insurance plans, the amount of actual responsibility assumed by providers is quite minimal. In these frameworks, providers agree to discounted charges, and sometimes to limitations on charges set by a specific dollar amount or by some specific charge-based index, and agree, in principle, to the legitimacy of the insurance company to review the consumption of care and to deny, retroactively, charges that may have been paid from inappropriately managed care. In these frameworks, the insurance company bears almost all of the responsibility for managing beneficiaries' care. The provider is merely a subcontractor who is paid according to what is billed and retains less charges as net revenues in instances where nonphysicians (the typical agents of the insurance company) "judge" the appropriateness of the care ordered and consumed.

Provider Autonomy

Many providers resent the fact that their actions are questioned by non-providers, many of whom are not physicians, and that providers who have relatively more expensive charges (e.g., emergency physicians, hospitals, ambulatory surgery centers, and surgeons) face more retrospective denials regardless of the appropriateness of the care that was consumed. To be sure, retrospective denials represent hindsight management, which is especially important for emergency department providers: Regardless of how care was managed *at the time it was incurred* (e.g., charges for services consumed by a patient who presents in the emergency department unconscious but who later turns out just to have fainted), charges for care consumed could be denied based on an outcome that might not have been positive had care been withheld.

The real issue here is that providers lose absolute autonomy under a managed care system where they assume little responsibility and therefore minimal risk. The fact that retrospective and retroactive denials occur with more regularity for the most expensive services points to a troubling pattern of rationing (see Chapter Four). From this perspective, the price that the risk bearer must pay for a given service becomes a determinant for its disallowance. After all, the services are being adjudicated by nonphysicians. On what basis can a nonphysician judge the appropriateness of a level of service directed by a physician?

Adversarial Relationships under the Current Paradigm

Nonphysicians can't judge what a physician does *except* by how much the services cost. The corollary is that less expensive services are allowed more frequently than more expensive services. While this type of rationing occurs quite frequently where providers assume little risk, I doubt that the risk bearer should be faulted. To be sure, the provider and the payor functions form an adversarial relationship: The provider wants to collect everything and the payor wants to pay nothing. The payor tells the provider only what must be reported as to why a decision (typically adverse) was made, but nothing of the available internal information that the payor had at its disposal (other than claim-type information that the provider was to supply) that was used to make the decision. On the other hand, the provider communicates with the payor only when money owed is overdue or when charges submitted were denied, but communicates nothing of the level of information (non-claim-related) that the payor should need to know to improve its decision-making capability.

I fail to see why this adversarial relationship should exist if both provider and payor have as their operating mission to provide high-quality service to an identified community! *The consumer always loses when rationing occurs,* especially when providers are adversarial in the protection of their monetary resources. The consumer (or enrollee) pays a premium for the expectation of quality service. Yet the payor has no means of determining quality service because the provider is not forthcoming in helping the payor make better decisions just to make sure that the payor's decisions that affect the provider are as favorable as possible, and only when such decisions need to be made. The sad fact is that the payors have never understood the nature of the providers' business, and the providers have been less than completely sensitive to the needs of the payors. Without the benefit of knowing how providers' decisions should ideally be made, the payors have found that their own decisions would have to be made based on the only information made available to them—price. The payors have taught the providers to ration on the basis of price alone.

At What Price Quality?

The rationing-based, price-sensitive relationship between payors and providers has undergone various transitions, which continue to sour the longer payors pay high costs and the longer providers shy away from assuming responsibility. In time, the question of quality arises. Quality is important for both medical and other, noninstitutional providers because their malpractice rates are tied to maintaining quality as a loss-prevention strategy. Quality is also important for general acute care hospitals, because the Joint Commission on Accreditation of Healthcare Organizations (JCAHO) requires quality measurement, quality assurance, and quality improvement as a continuing condition of certification (which, in most states, means the difference between remaining licensed or not). The impact of quality is lost on the general public, the insurance industry included, because the healthcare industry has been widely claiming that *all* doctors are of the highest quality and that *all* hospitals are of the highest quality. Here again, the public is not armed with the level of information necessary to help them distinguish between hospitals on the basis of quality care or quality service, beyond such minor issues as how much the hospital charges for aspirin or the appropriate taste and temperature of food it serves.

Providers who rely on outsiders to take fiscal responsibility for their patients' healthcare are now paying the awful price for all of those years of bad-faith misrepresentation of quality to the public. For example, the payor–provider relationship presupposes that quality exists (it's in both of their organizational missions) and that the payor should not have to pay extra for "quality" care. Without the means for distinguishing between different levels of care in the absolute sense, the payor can—sadly enough, in good faith—assume that the provider is acting in bad faith by charging for seemingly frivolous services. For example, why should an internist give every patient a Chem-20 (a single blood test that tests for

20 different blood characteristics) when some diagnoses might not specifically warrant any blood test or, perhaps, when a condition could have been diagnosed by a Chem-6? The payor isn't paying for the provider's malpractice insurance (which the payor would rightfully claim is part of the provider's overhead) and would have no way of understanding why it should pay for the provider's defensive medicine.

This elitism about quality is having profound implications for the responsibility of payors to pay for a differential level of care to ensure that quality occurs and for the very nature of the status quo as long as providers shun risk, give full care for polarized, at-risk consumers "entitled" to receive it, but ration care for the discriminated-against "nonentitled" consumers on the basis of price alone.

THE IMPORTANCE OF MANAGED CARE

Management involves assuming responsibility. Providers have responsibility for the medical and/or nonmedical care of their patients. "Quality" providers manage the way care is consumed so as to provide appropriate depth and breadth of care in a way that yields the best outcomes and, it is hoped, in turn, the highest levels of consumer satisfaction. Managed care does not detract from this scheme but instead injects a level of accountability that identifies who rightfully assumes the responsibility for well-managed care (and enjoys the benefits thereof) and who rightfully assumes the responsibility for poorly managed care (and suffers *all* of the consequences thereof).

Finally, the paradigm of managed care espoused by this book involves the process of proper management under capitation, the opportunities presented by capitation that are ignored or unrealized within the current healthcare environment, and the strategies by which nonprovider enterprises dependent on the healthcare industry (particularly those whose incomes are 50 percent or more attributable to this healthcare industry) can survive and flourish in an era where capitated managed care becomes the dominant payor source for the healthcare industry.

Chapter Two

Leveling the Playing Field: Speaking the Right Language

One of the problems with the field of managed care in our society is the use of jargon. The use of jargon in the healthcare delivery system originated with physicians and continued with nurses and various other allied health professionals. In our industry, jargon connotes that there is specialized understanding not known to the layperson. Frequently, this jargon involves abbreviations and acronyms. The use of jargon by clinicians has damaged our industry in the eyes of the public, connoting an aloofness that transcends even to our language.

The use of jargon by clinicians also serves to polarize workers in healthcare settings according to "those who know" and "those who don't know." Nonclinicians who work with, or manage, clinicians try to learn their jargon. In addition, the nonclinicians introduce their own jargon, which bewilders and confuses clinicians, who are frequently unaware of the extent and amount of jargon they routinely use. As a result, "those who don't know" give others the impression that "they do know" by using jargon and the newest phrases, whether they truly understand them or not. The result is a workplace where jargon is used quite commonly, but the terms have different meanings according to the level of factual knowledge their users have.

Jargon proliferates in general acute care hospital settings, but it is not limited to such workplaces. Hospitals are host to both intradisciplinary jargon—such as how surgical registered nurses in the operating room might refer to different cases, certain physicians, or certain procedures—and interdisciplinary jargon—such as a payor classification (like "Medi-Medi," which refers to a patient who is covered by both Medicare and Medicaid), a patient classification, or a level of patient acuity (such as an unconscious patient with a "positive Q-sign," characterized by an open mouth with the patient's tongue hanging out). Jargon also exists in settings where there is more than one provider, whether in a hospital or some other place or organization where providers practice; such settings include physicians' offices, clinics, long-term care facilities, and behavioral health settings (both inpatient and outpatient).

The field of managed care has introduced an entirely new level and kind of jargon into the healthcare industry. Because managed care started with insurance companies looking for different payment mechanisms in hospital settings, clinicians were "out of the jargon loop" from the outset. For much of the early years of managed care, the insurance industry jargon was shared only with the setting's senior managers and typically with a manager of contracting, who emanates most commonly from the insurance industry but most recently from managed care organization settings. As managed care moves more of a setting's business away from reimbursement and toward prospective payment, including capitation, the pressure to redefine and reengineer clinical processes increases, thus bringing greater numbers of employees in contact with managed care jargon.

One of the problems with such a progression of jargon exposure in healthcare settings is that the dynamics of a marketplace's maturity in managed care will influence the extent to which the jargon of managed care becomes part of the vocabulary of physicians and clinicians. Markets such as Northern Minnesota and Southern California are very mature managed care markets, while many parts of New England and the Southern United States typify very immature managed care markets. For example, someone in New England or the South may hear terms like *POS, capitation,* and *MSO* from colleagues in Southern California, or read articles in journals written by professionals from more mature managed care markets. Sometimes these terms are defined, but many times the definitions reflect the level of understanding of the user, not a definitive source (in part because there are few definitive sources yet recognized in this emerging field). Ego plays a large part in this misunderstanding as well.

The function of ego in preventing acknowledgment of unfamiliarity with or discomfort in using jargon is particularly crippling in the healthcare industry. Perhaps this ego stems from nonclinicians' resentment toward clinicians (and others) who use jargon to exclude them from conversations; the nonclinicians consciously or unconsciously retaliate by injecting their own form of jargon into conversations with clinicians. The crippling aspect is that members of the healthcare industry don't typically ask what new terms mean at the time they are spoken. They will usually just nod their heads or convey the impression that they understand the terms when, in fact, their level of knowledge is far from complete. In this manner they themselves will often use the terms among their colleagues and among middle and senior managers who use the terminology more often. Because of the function of ego, managers might wonder to themselves how a clinician can know so much about certain esoteric managed care terms yet might not question whether the clinician really understands the term.

We are also seeing a "cross-contamination" of language, particularly managed care terms that may have entered certain work settings as jargon, among both clinicians and nonclinicians throughout the United States, and to a limited extent (as of this writing) throughout the world. What should have been a renaissance of language that finally bridged the health and insurance industries has devolved into a modern form of the Tower of Babel. People use the same words, but the effect is greater confusion rather than greater understanding. This new Tower of Babel occurs in an egocentric healthcare industry, whose members' sense of self-worth is so damaged that they perceive they are unable to acknowledge matters or terms they don't truly understand.

The cross-contamination also occurs because the healthcare industry remains quite nepotistic. One result of continuing education requirements for physicians, nurses, other healthcare clinicians, and even administrative staff aligned with professional organizations (e.g., the American College of Healthcare Executives for CEOs and COOs; the Healthcare Financial Management Association for CFOs and other financially oriented professions; the Healthcare Information Management and Systems Society for CIOs and other computer-oriented professionals; the Medical Group Management Association; and the American Guild of Patient Account Managers) is that tremendous networking occurs in the healthcare industry. Most everyone knows, has heard, or has worked with most everyone else.

While this nepotism can make circles of professionals seem like a country club and can make penetration by outsiders or newcomers seem formidable, there is a significant upside: word of mouth is a valuable catalyst for change. If a new program, approach, service, method, or product works in one part of the country, professionals within the same niche in the healthcare industry are soon trying it too. Word travels especially fast in the 1990s, with such implements as the Internet, E-mail, commercial online services and chat lines, and even electronic bulletin board services sponsored by professional organizations themselves (e.g., the Healthcare Financial Management Association's "HFMA-Net," available at no fee to the association's 33,000 members). The nepotism and cross-contamination observed in the healthcare industry do not seem to be segmented among private- and public-sector professionals; hence, physicians receiving salaries from county departments of health services (public sector) hang out at the same continuing education and advocacy meetings as their private-sector counterparts. The major difference is not the sites where professionals congregate, but how each sector understands the same information given at any single site.

PRIVATE- VERSUS PUBLIC-SECTOR DISTINCTIONS IN UNDERSTANDING TERMINOLOGY

The confounding cross-contamination of industry jargon is particularly acute in the public health sector. The most basic discrepancy involves the term *managed care*. Here's how the problem is created: A top official of a local health department is a member of a professional organization such as the American College of Healthcare Executives (ACHE). This official attends an ACHE meeting, such as an annual national conference, and hears private-sector speakers talking about how they've responded to managed care in their facility, agency, or operation. Even if the speakers define the term *managed care,* the official will likely hear a different definition of the term at each session because there is no standard lexicon, so far, in this industry and egos are usually so high that no single individual is willing to concede that he or she may have misunderstood the basic concept. A reverse scenario occurs when members of the private sector attend a meeting or session frequented primarily by public-sector professionals. In short, the basic problem in defining the term *managed care* is that it is understood differently within each sector.

Private Sector Understanding of Managed Care

The private sector tends to define the term *managed care* as an idiom in that its definition is completely unrelated to *care* and largely unrelated to *management.* A fairly authoritative private-sector definition of the term is the same as the one given in Chapter One: *Managed care is a means of providing healthcare services within a defined network of healthcare providers who are given the responsibility to manage and provide high-quality, cost-effective healthcare.* A private-sector nuance is that giving providers the responsibility to manage is not the same as actually allowing them to manage. While the "responsibility to manage" may be delegated via a managed care contract of sorts, the infrastructure within which management can occur is often neglected and/or unspecified. Three implications of this compromised infrastructure are as follows: (1) Providers are not given the basic information they need to manage a population; (2) Providers are not given the means to manage such information (were such information available to the providers and/or were the providers to know that they need a level of information beyond the level given to them), in terms of technology, manpower, and sophistication; and (3) Providers are unaware of all their responsibilities—whether specific, inferred, or implied—in order to provide quality healthcare to populations included within such managed care. Because providers receive so little useful information to implement true management, and because they are well aware of the financial risks and obligations they assume in entering into managed care contracts, *the only option available to them is to ration.* This statement is very strong and merits some clarification.

Rationing As a Management Strategy of Last Resort

Let's say I am the administrator of a medical group that has been contracted to provide high-quality, cost-effective healthcare offered by a health plan to a particular population. I know from my managed care contract what my financial obligations are (e.g., that I'm willing to accept a discounted fee-for-service that represents 75 percent of usual and customary rates and that the health plan will give me a substantial financial incentive to reduce my group's overall healthcare expenditures), and I understand the various financial trade-offs: what I receive if my group is successful at managing care and what I give up if my group is less than successful. I also understand how little the health plan will do from the moment I sign the contract and that I accept a greater level of responsibility up to certain dollar thresholds for each member of the managed care population I'll be serving.

While I know that I will be financially responsible for this population and understand the consequences of such financial responsibility on both the upside and the downside, I know nothing about how I can manage this population within the given financial constraints. Indeed, I know next to nothing about the population for whom I have financial responsibility: I have medical records only for those members of the population who have consumed healthcare services (whether in a doctor's office, in another ambulatory setting, or as an inpatient) and have no computerized records, except perhaps for billing and collections information, which record only the level of information needed to receive money for a billed claim. I might not even have a computer, or an appropriate level of computerized sophistication (hardware and software) to make sense of such data if I had them; and even if I had computerized billing information, I'd have very little useful data to assist me in real management. I wouldn't know which members of my population are current or behind on immunizations (including tetanus boosters), which members are most at risk for preventable medical conditions, which members are most at risk for unpreventable medical conditions (which will cost me money), and which members of the population are healthy enough that they likely won't require any healthcare at all. In short, my group is set up to be surprised and to be injured financially from the surprises. As such, I have no means by which to manage my population, to allocate my scarce resources effectively, to plan how to manage my population better, or to assess what level of financial losses this population will create for my group.

   Therefore, the only strategy I have available to me, in order to maximize my group's finances under this managed care contract whereby I lose money for each occurrence of consumptive behavior—whether or not it is appropriate—is to reduce my overall consumption whether or not it is appropriate to do so. My strategies would include shortening my hours of operation, eliminating weekend and holiday hours of service, reducing operating expenses (including staffing), reducing capital expenditures, and cutting back on PBX expenses by installing voice mail. (It is not surprising to be calling in to voice mail systems in so many medical groups and IPAs that have signed managed care contracts, particularly capitated contracts.)

   If I adopt a rationing-oriented approach to managed care, my operational focus might change as well. I might therefore consider any member contact to be a negative contact, especially if allowing such contact would have a certain negative financial consequence and only an uncertain negative quality consequence. Taking this approach to the ultimate level (hypothetically speaking, and not to suggest that this strategy exists to a widespread degree), I might install voice mail with the expressed intent of discouraging my employees from returning all but the most urgent member phone calls (since the call was placed to initiate a consumption of healthcare service and not returning the call would eliminate a less-than-clearly appropriate consumptive contact) by creating user-unfriendly menuing systems to discourage all but the most tenacious consumers from leaving a message in the first place. In short, I'd have financial disincentives for consumptive behaviors on the part of the population for whom I'm financially responsible, but no means to distinguish between truly appropriate and inappropriate consumptive behavior. In other words, I am inadvertently challenged and operationally straitjacketed to manage the population in a quality-conscious manner, if at all, and have financial disincentives for each incident of healthcare consumptive actions. As the chief manager for this group, I'd be left to manage only what I can manage, even though the act of doing so is nothing short of rationing. My rationing actions would represent all that I am able to do; they would not represent a malicious intent to cheat my members or to downgrade the level of quality and value they might derive from my physicians. Yet the term *managed care,* from a private-sector perspective, still incorporates marketing terms like *quality, care,* and *management,* which are largely unpracticed among medical groups and IPAs involved in managed care contracts.

Private-Sector Managed Care versus Minimized Cost

Thus, from the private sector's standpoint, the act of managing care is an act of controlling costs. Because so few healthcare providers have any true form of cost accounting (beyond a typical "guesstimate" of an overall ratio of Medicare-reported costs and actual, or billed, charges), the actual management of costs involves the minimization of costs. This operational definition of managed care is a far cry from such elements as quality (which is largely ignored on anything smaller than a global or community level), appropriate care (indistinguishable from the unnecessary incurring of costs), and management (which relies on a level of information neither collected, shared, nor maintained). This notion of minimized cost being a private-sector understanding of the term *managed care* is antithetical to the public sector's understanding of the same term.

Public-Sector Managed Care

The public sector approaches the concept of managed care much differently from the private sector, almost suggesting that emissaries of the public sector in private-sector circles have incorporated the term into the lexicon of the public sector before truly understanding how the private sector defines and uses it. Nevertheless, the term *managed care* is used in the public sector to contemporize its long-standing efforts to mobilize needed healthcare services and interventions in improving the care of underserved populations. Just as I equate the private sector's definition of managed care with the term *minimized cost,* I equate the public sector's definition of managed care with the concept of *managed caring.*

To understand the public sector's perspective in approaching the concept of managed care, one must understand how the public sector sees its healthcare world. The public sector views itself as a safety net for the have-nots of our society: the medically needy or medically vulnerable who lack the financial resources to seek the best care and protection. In order to add value to these populations, the public sector, especially so among state and city/county healthcare agencies, seeks to improve the level of medical resources made available to them matched with a level of documentation to assure that such individuals do not fall through the cracks.

In the process of managing care, public-sector providers have been adding value and enhancing and documenting the quality of healthcare services offered to their clients for some time now. It is interesting to note that the public sector has been attempting to improve, and in some cases has succeeded, the operational processes in providing care to its members. This process improvement came at a time when the private sector was still wrestling with the philosophical concept of healthcare quality and its definition within the industry (a concept that even today lacks a gold-standard definition within the healthcare industry aside from different operational definitions utilized by certain payors and providers).

The assumption within the public sector is that public health populations will be poorly served or underserved unless their care is more appropriately managed by responsible public-sector providers and agencies. Thus, the public sector defines managed care in purely operational terms while the private sector defines managed care in purely financial terms. Although this book will deal largely with private-sector managed care issues and implications, the public sector has much to learn, as few people within the public organizations truly understand the language of the private sector. I believe that managed care can work only if the private and public sectors join forces to mobilize cost-effective and quality-appropriate strategies and solutions. Distinctions and untapped opportunities like these must be understood when making generalized statements about managed care and emerging managed care paradigms and models.

MANAGED CARE MODELS

The healthcare delivery system in the United States is moving rapidly toward managed care and eventually toward capitated managed care. It is my belief that the payor side of the industry is responsible for transforming the healthcare market to capitated managed care (see Chapter Three), a process that involves creating the models and infrastructures that could eventually allow capitation to occur. As a result, the market could not possibly move to capitation unless a plan and certain levels of groundwork are firmly established.

Integrated Models

One level of groundwork to be established in the move to capitation involves creating payor models that could thrive under capitation; at a more preemptive level, payors could encourage only those provider models that would function best within such payor models while discouraging those provider models that compromise or effectively challenge such payor strategies. The discussion of models is itself insidious, because frequently it is the payor organizations more so than medical provider organizations that do the required amount of strategic planning to influence organizational design issues. While general acute care hospitals and managed care organizations do a fair amount of planning as well, they are often restricted in their ability to create or change medical provider organizational models short of creating risk-assumptive structures like syndications, initial public offerings, venture capital corporations, and physician-hospital organizations (PHOs).

Furthermore, integrated models reflect the paradigm shifts occurring or not occurring within the marketplace. For example, just as institutional providers did not change from a reimbursement-dependent model to a prospective management model when the government adopted the prospective payment system (refer back to the discussion of DRGs in

Chapter One), neither did medical provider organizations. To be sure, independent practice associations (IPAs—one provider model particularly pervasive in the public sector) are organized according to the reimbursement nature of the past: Providers create claims, in most cases processed internally through a central IPA office, and are *reimbursed* according to the claims for which they bill; the claims-based system remains intact even as the IPA office receives income through capitated arrangements between a health plan and the IPA as a whole. As a structure, therefore, an IPA is more at home with reimbursement-based compensation, and physician members of IPAs participating in capitated managed care are themselves insulated from capitated risk, instead continuing to be compensated according to billed claims.

The move toward integrated models involves coordination between interested parties. One integrated model, the administrative-service-only or administrative services organization (both definitions are used for the abbreviation ASO), seeks to collect a portion of capitation made available by an HMO on the premise that this portion is a headache that providers don't wish, or are unable, to absorb. Administrative service represents the infrastructural needs of filing claims and maintaining claims data, utilization review and management, adjudication services, coordinating benefits, billing members for co-payments, collecting customer satisfaction data (as providers may now, and hopefully will all soon, request), and possibly even scheduling services. ASO fees command up to 7 to 12 percent of the capitation premium, more if the HMO contracts directly with an independent ASO or an ASO product within an MSO (see below), less if the HMO adds provider capitation for the assumption of this additional responsibility, and even less if the provider accepts the higher capitation and then subcontracts with an ASO on a subcapitated arrangement. Yet the members of the healthcare industry best reacting to changes in the marketplace are the ones who are shaping the marketplace: the payors.

Payor Models

The two primary payor models in our healthcare delivery system are HMOs and PPOs. Contrary to popular belief, prepaid group practices (the forerunners of HMOs) predated PPOs, even though PPOs are a less restrictive payor model. In an HMO, a member pays a premium for coverage (typically for the member and his or her dependents). In return for the premium, the member selects a gatekeeper physician from among a list of physicians who make up the HMO staff, panel, or group (see the section labeled "Provider Models" on page 34); how that patient is managed depends on the specific provider model. A member who actually goes to an HMO physician receives no bill and pays a minor co-payment at time of service (from $2 to $20, but most typically about $5) that is not tied to consumption-based charges. A member who requires services of an HMO facility (whether clinic, general acute care hospital, or home care) pays a less minor, but still not consumption-based, co-payment, the amount of which depends on whether such services were directed by the gatekeeper, directed by another plan physician (who is not the gatekeeper), or self-directed by the member (such as going to a hospital's emergency department). A member who seeks medical care outside the HMO (whether for primary care—general or family medicine, internal medicine, or pediatrics—not done by the designated gatekeeper or for outside specialty care) is typically not covered as part of the premium; in such cases, members themselves pay for all such charges incurred with no reimbursement required by the HMO.

HMO products, especially in a capitated form, are hugely profitable for HMOs. Medicare Risk HMO products, always provided via capitation, are substantially more profitable for HMOs. Because of HCFA requirements, HMOs can't sell Medicare Risk products unless there is an adequate base of commercial (non-Medicare, non-indigent, and otherwise unspecialized) capitated lives. The Health Care Financing Administration currently defines an *adequate base* of commercial lives as comprising no less than 50 percent of the total Medicare covered lives. Therefore, if an HMO wished to sell a Medicare Risk product, it could sell only as many Medicare Risk premiums as it had commercial-paid premiums. For example, if the HMO receives approval from HCFA to offer 100,000 senior households in a given market coverage in a federally qualified Medicare Risk product, the HMO must demonstrate to HCFA that no fewer than 100,000 subscriptions are in place for a federally qualified commercial capitation product. Only Southern California's United Health Plan (UHP) remains as having received a waiver to offer Medicare Risk without a 50 percent coverage by commercial capitated lives; the other waiver recipient was South Florida's International Medical Centers (IMC), which has since gone out of business. Applications for new waivers are now being considered by HCFA.

The other primary payor model is a preferred provider organization (PPO). PPOs are not yet true players in the managed care marketplace because they assume no real risk, do not involve managed care in anything other than a retrospective basis and the requirement of second opinions for key medical and surgical diagnoses, and are virtually indistinguishable from reimbursement methodologies such as discounted fee-for-service.

Discounted fee-for-service must be understood in comparison with the fee-for-service methodology. In a fee-for-service reimbursement methodology, a provider submits a claim to a payor for a particular set of consumed services. The payor pays the provider a reimbursement fee based on what charges were generated and whether such charges were consistent with the usual and customary rate (UCR) for that area. Unbelievable as it sounds, there is no such thing as a definable UCR for any area because this rate is self-regulated by the insurance industry. As such, there are no objective standards for how UCRs are to be determined and indexed, for how often they need to be updated, or for determining if a UCR needs to be changed. In the minds of providers, UCRs appear to represent what a payor chooses to pay for any single occurrence of charges. A typical reimbursement methodology under group insurance and private insurance plans that still use fee-for-service is to cover 80 percent of UCR-based charges, with the remaining 20 percent of charges the financial responsibility of the insured, after satisfaction of the appropriate deductible—which makes the insured responsible for the first dollar threshold of billed charges, typically $250 to $500, but as much as $1,000 to $2,000 in "expensive" healthcare markets such as Southern California, where such group insurance plans have tried to keep premium prices "affordable."

In a discounted fee-for-service (DFFS) reimbursement methodology, by contrast, the amount of coverage is a discount off of the UCR, which is negotiated directly with the providers. Any charges incurred that exceed the discounted UCR are part of the co-payment paid by the insured, in addition to deductibles. The insured will not be told what the discount level and what the UCR are; rather, he or she will receive an itemization that shows the percentage of "allowed" and "disallowed" charges for which he or she is financially responsible. Most group insurance plans today use the DFFS arrangement, including many HMOs that do not yet use capitated payments to providers. In DFFS, the typical ratio of coverage is still 80 percent off the discounted UCR, with the remaining 20 percent of the discounted UCR and all disallowed charges the responsibility of the insured.

In PPOs, the insured pays a premium to the preferred provider organization. In return for the premium paid, the insured is "encouraged" to seek care from a list of providers who agree to abide by the provisions of the PPO. The "preferred provider" accepts a typically deeper discount than under DFFS, operationalized by the PPO giving the provider a "price list" by current procedural terminology (CPT) code. This price list governs what the provider will charge; hence, every provider charge that conforms to the current price list is "allowable." The current price list is nothing more than a definitive listing of the "dollar effects" of discounted fee-for-service; in other words, the provider might agree to a $75 charge for a limited exam of an established patient, rather than a 75 percent discount off of a $100 UCR for the same diagnostic service (itemized by its CPT code). It is also a cleaner agreement from the PPO's standpoint, in that a subsequent adjustment to the price list might indicate that the allowable charge is now $70, instead of having to account for what the "new" UCR is and what the "new" discount ratio is for the same procedure.

Under a PPO, the provider also agrees to utilization review (UR), whereby a separate department or subcontracted agency ensures that the provider sought preauthorizations for services or treatments that the PPO determines require such permission. These UR studies are done on the basis of claims submitted for payment and are therefore retrospective in nature. Providers are not limited in how many PPOs they can "contract" with, and they are driven by the premise that PPOs will give them added volume of insureds to offset the deeper discounts in what they agree to charge. Our experience has shown that many physicians and hospitals have signed up with every PPO in the marketplace that will allow them to contract, with very few providers in capitated markets seeing PPOs as a majority of their payor mix.

From the consumer side of PPOs, the distinction between PPOs and DFFS is even less distinct. Insureds who seek medical care from a preferred provider typically have 90 percent (instead of 80 percent under DFFS) of their charges covered, meaning that their co-payment is "only" 10 percent of allowable billed charges (instead of 20 percent under DFFS). Insureds who seek medical care outside the PPO are covered for half of their charges or less; a typical ratio is 40 percent coverage of all billed charges (akin to nondiscounted fee-for-service) outside the PPO. Thus, under a PPO system, the consumer still retains the right to have free choice of providers but the privilege comes with a hefty price tag if care is sought outside the preferred provider organization.

From both a consumer and provider standpoint, there is very little about PPOs that legitimately qualifies as managed care. PPOs provide a layer of profit to the business by encouraging providers to accept below-market prices and charging significant "penalties" for members seeking care outside the panel. The PPOs bear no risk for having inadequate specialty coverage on their panels; indeed, having only one or two physicians representing key specialties like OB/GYN, cardiology, and orthopedics increases the probability (and perhaps profitability) of members seeking care outside the PPO. A staff model HMO (see below), by contrast, bears the risk for inadequate specialty coverage by forcing primary care physicians to hold on to higher acuity patients who otherwise require specialty care, thus having negative effects on consumer satisfaction and consumer wellness. While immature capitated markets are quick to include PPO utilization with HMO utilization and call the sum managed care, the reality is that PPOs are no more part of managed care than are group or private insurance plans that make use of a DFFS reimbursement methodology. The only legitimate managed care entity of the two is clearly the HMO, which is hungry for market share.

Two other popular payor models, exclusive provider organizations (EPOs) and point-of-service plans (POS plans or PSPs), are more related to HMO sales than they are to PPOs (see below). A third new model, accountable health plans (AHPs), seeks to differentiate PPOs to compete better with HMOs. AHPs now emerging seek to create gatekeepers among primary care members of preferred provider lists and to require gatekeeper approval for specialty medical and institutional care, while still allowing insureds to seek care outside the PPO, albeit for a larger penalty (e.g., coverage for only 25 to 33 percent of billed charges). Other AHP products coming to market include hybrids of flexible spending accounts that still provide for freedom of choice but put the consumer at risk for consumption of services above certain dollar thresholds.

The EPO and PSP models differ in terms of who is solicited to improve HMO sales. The EPO is targeted to an employer, and the PSP is targeted to a provider. These models are seemingly offered for extended subscriptions, but in practice they are designed to drive incremental HMO sales within one to two years. They both prey on an inherent unwillingness on the part of the consumer to purchase or belong to an HMO-based plan.

An EPO would be targeted to an employer (usually a benefits coordinator in the company's human resources department) that has misgivings about changing the company's benefit package to include an HMO, often at the expense of group insurance plans that give employees unlimited choice at hefty premium or co-payment levels. Some employers feel that offering HMO choices may signal to employees that the era of managed care has arrived at their company. In the 1990s, however, the stigma associated with most HMOs has eased, but misgivings and distrust remain.

In an attempt to attract a distrustful employer, the HMO account executive would indicate the availability of an EPO plan that is more like a trusted PPO than a distrusted HMO. Under the EPO, the account executive might say, employees would be able to "sample" the physicians who are part of the HMO panel, would pay a small co-payment (like the $5 co-payments of HMO plans) when consuming care under the EPO, but would be free to seek medical care outside the EPO panel with a penalty (e.g., 25 percent coverage of billed charges). To the untrained eye of the benefit coordinator, the EPO appears to be very similar to a PPO, except that the members of the preferred panel are more accomplished managed care physicians than those who typically populate a preferred provider organization. What is missed on the front end is the risk of employees developing doctor–patient relationships with "rented" physicians, a bonding that might otherwise force a longer-term relationship with the HMO than if the employer had no such encumbrances. The enticement is sweetened with premium pricing that is higher than HMO premiums but significantly less than PPO and group insurance rates, all locked in for about a year.

What might be missed on the front end is quite obvious on the back end. After a year of employees sampling the HMO panel while subscribing to the EPO, the HMO account executive has a very different meeting with the benefits coordinator. The encounter usually begins with something like "I have good news and bad news." The bad news is invariably that losses incurred by the HMO with its EPO products over the last 12 months have, regretfully, required the HMO to raise next year's premiums for the EPO quite substantially—in some cases as much as a 100 percent premium increase. The good news is usually that the excellent medical-loss experience (total medical claims paid as a percentage of total premium collected) of the HMO product has allowed for only a marginal premium increase over last year, but overall lower than the EPO premium paid over the prior period. Employers who don't get the message after the first year will usually pay outrageous rates the second year, and even higher rates each subsequent year until they either drop EPO coverage or convert to HMO coverage. In fact, the longer employers who opt for "teaser" EPO coverage resist paying for HMO coverage, the higher the HMO premiums they'll be paying, if allowed at all.

A point-of-service-based payor plan is geared to providers, typically physicians in immature capitation markets, who are subject to a plight similar to that of the benefits coordinator but with more disastrous effects for holding out. In mature capitation markets, by contrast, PSPs are used to improve the marketability of staff model HMOs (see below) by giving members added choice, thereby influencing new sales and member retention. A provider relations liaison from the HMO visits a physician, typically a primary care physician practicing in an immature capitation market. The liaison invites the physician to join the already-forming HMO panel, group, or staff. The physician responds that he or she is hesitant about joining an HMO, based on rumors or on a reluctance to be part of a panel with a key doctor or two who, the physician might have heard, practices substandard medicine, or is difficult to work with, or is a foreign medical graduate, and so on. The provider relations liaison indicates that the HMO is so willing to have the physician join that it will extend an invitation for the physician to join its point-of-service plan.

By belonging to the POS plan, the physician will be able to "sample" the HMO panel without being required to practice exclusively within it. In return, the HMO will direct POS plan patients to the physician at the physician's current office; the physician will be paid on a DFFS basis and is free to continue seeing other patients outside the POS plan as desired. During the period, the physician will submit claims data and be subject to utilization management processes, commensurate with most PPOs and the few HMOs that are in that market. After the period, assuming there is continued interest on the part of the HMO and if space is still available, the provider relations liaison will again invite the physician to join the HMO. To the untrained eye, the physician on the fence can experience the HMO panel firsthand, kick the tires, and determine if he or she could enjoy or tolerate working for the HMO on a more full-time basis, all with no strings attached and without any coercion to change practice behaviors and referral relationships. To the trained eye, however, the HMO is watching very carefully.

After six months to one year of being part of a POS plan, especially in emerging capitated markets that are successful in filling HMO panels quickly (much more so in the mid-1990s than in the early 1990s and late 1980s), few physicians are invited to convert to the HMO panel. Those who are allowed to join are invariably excluded from receiving capitated rates initially, a period of time when capitation rates are the highest and when those physicians who receive the earliest capitations are more able to generate subcapitation contracts than those who receive capitation in the third and fourth years. Almost no physicians are lucky enough to be part of a POS plan for more than one year.

On the surface, this low conversion rate might seem like failing to make partner in a law firm or not being offered a job after a second interview. In reality, a year on a POS plan can very easily drive a physician to bankruptcy. Here's how it works: A family practitioner working 60 hours a week agrees to be part of a POS panel. The physician, going in, might have had a payor mix that was 30 percent Medicare, 10 percent Medicaid, 10 percent PPO, and 50 percent group insurance. Because the physician is already working a 60-hour week, the physician is unable to expand the amount of hours worked unless additional physicians and/or extenders are hired; since the physician views the slow move to the HMO as a step toward retirement, this family practitioner mistakenly perceives that the POS plan will allow him or her to cut back hours worked instead of expand them. In addition, the physician is more thrifty in terms of what is spent for managed care business. By the end of the year, assuming the 60-hour work week was maintained, the physician's payor mix might now be 40 percent POS (paid on DFFS, like group insurance), 30 percent Medicare, 10 percent Medicaid, 10 percent PPO, and 10 percent group insurance (also paid on DFFS). Because both group insurance and POS pay via DFFS, the physician might experience no reduction of profitability with this changed payor mix during this one-year sampling. At this point, the provider relations liaison would likely not invite the physician to join the HMO (unless the physician was self-taught in effective managed care medicine techniques), would almost definitely not invite the physician to continue with the POS plan, or, if joining the HMO is a possibility, might offer a payment structure that is much less generous than DFFS and possibly extend capitation or subcapitation rates that are on the lower side of the market. If the physician chooses, or is forced, to leave the POS plan without replacement HMO business, insolvency is a real possibility.

Because the family practitioner did not work additional hours, and because this physician allowed the POS business to replace valuable group insurance business, the physician effectively loses 80 percent of his or her business when walking away from the POS plan at the end of the trial year (the 40 percent POS business when walking away and the 40 percent group insurance business that the physician didn't realize he or she was losing over the year that he or she was seeing replacement POS patients). More insidiously, the physician was unable to retain the group insurance business—which is typically the case—because the physician was too busy to cater to this "product line" by giving preferential and same-day appointments, keeping waiting times low, and having office staff do much of the paperwork for the patient as a convenience. Group insurance patients, who know they are "cream" business and expect to be treated that way, invariably leave the offices of POS physicians and become patients of competitor private-practice physicians. Once such ex-POS physicians realize that 40 percent of their business has evaporated and that the other 40 percent can't quickly be replaced, and that it's the cream business that has defected, the physicians are usually unable to reclaim the business they lost, all in an era where group insurance business covers groups with large books of business that involve substantial deductions from revenue (like Medicare, Medicaid, and some PPOs). While the net loss was only 40 percent, the effect on the provider is an 80 percent loss.

To the consumer, the POS plan seems similar to the EPO. The insured pays minimal co-payments when seeing panel physicians, and still retains the right to see nonpanel physicians, albeit at a 75 to 80 percent coverage penalty. There is also a fair possibility that an insured's private practice physician might turn up as part of the POS panel, for as long as the physician is part of the POS plan. Many don't realize that physicians joining a POS plan and cutting back hours (most typically hurting the business they shouldn't be hurting) are actually headed for early retirement anyway.

Provider Models

There are three types of payor models that have implications for medical and institutional providers under capitated managed care: the staff model, the panel model, and the group model. These are HMO models, created by payors, that have implications for how capitation is paid and how capitation funds are managed at the provider level. As one might expect, there is a natural intertwining between provider and payor interests when considering these models.

Literally the first payor model for HMOs is the staff-model HMO. Originated by Kaiser Permanente and adapted by other health plans, the staff model is probably the most efficient structure for managing the health of capitated populations and maintaining appropriate levels of information to manage care effectively. The staff model locates all of the facets of an entire healthcare delivery system within close proximity of one another and unifies the control of the system's infrastructure. Approximately 10 percent of all HMOs in current operation use the staff model.

At FHP's headquarters in Fountain Valley, California, which up until mid-1995 was the site of FHP's only remaining staff-model program, the company has had its own hospital located in close proximity to its administrative offices, a long-term care facility, a clinic, an owned pharmacy, and medical offices; while some of the administrative and medical offices are off-campus, most are located within a short walk of one another and free campus transportation—including to and from parking areas—is provided by a tram. Each of the campus locales is tied in to the same computer system, and dedicated staff in the administrative offices use utilization and member demographic data to predict resource consumption and program services accordingly. Similar models are used by Kaiser Permanente and other staff-model HMOs.

The downsides to staff-model HMOs explain why they generate the lowest relative market share among health plans. One downside to the staff-model HMO is that the consumer has no real or perceived provider choices outside the static staff. The staff model is entirely flexible in extending levels of real choice within its own constraints (e.g., members are legitimately able to see any provider at any time, and to go to any hospital at any time—as long as the providers and hospitals are part of the staff-model HMO). Unfortunately, other payor models afford their members with greater levels of perceived choice (but not significantly different real choice) than is available within staff-model HMOs. A potential hedge by staff-model HMOs like Kaiser Permanente is the creation of a point-of-service option (see above), which allows its members to seek medical care with POS-affiliated physicians who are not members of Kaiser Permanente Medical Group; the trade-off is that members pay higher co-payments for this added level of choice, a trade-off that might allow Kaiser to regain market share lost to its non-staff-model competitors, once the POS option is more widely marketed and promoted within its medical trade areas.

The most significant downside is that staff-model HMOs are virtually locked out of new market expansions. The reason for this downside reality is that staff-model HMOs control all aspects of their operation, resulting in an unwieldy infrastructure. Say, for example, that a staff-model HMO based in Fountain Valley, California, recognized a new market opportunity for managed care in Shelby County, Georgia. Under a staff-model system, the HMO would have to build or purchase an entire hospital; employ physicians (or develop various PHOs, discussed in more detail below) to be housed adjacent to the hospital (probably involving either new construction or purchase of an existing medical office building that can be ripped off of its foundation, transported to a site adjacent to the hospital, and placed in that location), whether or not there are any patients; build and stock an entire pharmacy within the same physical location as the physicians and hospital, regardless of the number of members; and so on. This entire infrastructure, clearly not financially feasible, needs to be created at the outset before any potential members can be solicited and subscriptions generated. Such an infrastructure would have to be created based solely on a calculated risk that such a market exists in Shelby County in the first place. The staff model is at its best when such markets do exist and when customers prefer staff-model HMO care to other forms; the staff model is at its worst when such ready-made markets do not yet exist and the exorbitant ramp-up costs of initiating a pure staff-model HMO make it unable to compete in new markets.

The panel-model HMO was the alternative chosen by FHP to compete more effectively in new markets. Rather than replicate an entire staff-model infrastructure in order to respond to market opportunities, FHP was able to enter into loose contractual relationships with a local hospital and a ready-made (or last-minute-created, in many cases) panel of physicians and other clinicians mobilized and motivated to take care of the institutional and medical needs, respectively, of a block of members residing within that general area. The most universally known form of physician panel is the independent practice association structure known as an IPA.

An IPA is a "virtual" organization of primary- and specialty-care physicians who might not know one another or even practice in geographically homogeneous locations. Individual physicians may belong to several IPAs, none of which restricts a physician's style of practice or demands conformity to too many financial, clinical, quality, or even interpersonal requirements. Members of IPAs run their own operations as they see fit, and the IPA itself exerts very little control outside the scope of individual managed care contracts. Each contract for which the IPA may negotiate on behalf of its members represents a different, loose affiliation of medical providers who are contractually united on paper (or, more accurately, in cyberspace) alone. As previously stated, the IPA may negotiate a capitated rate with a payor (whether a health plan directly or other medical providers on a specific, subcontracted basis—a payment mechanism known as *subcapitation*), but compensates its member physicians on the basis of internally managed, billed claims. The capitated rate, and the levels of risk imposed by such rates, do not trickle down to the IPA physician; rather, the member physician is compensated via more traditional payment mechanisms like discounted fee-for-service.

The IPA model is relatively easy to create and relatively easy for a health plan to manage, in that there is a single point of contact for the entire IPA. The IPA's administrator is the accountable representative of the physician members of the IPA to the health plans and providers that generate its revenue streams. In addition, an IPA is relatively simple to organize; medical panels have been created in the past in just hours, sometimes by hospitals so desperate to negotiate for managed care contracts that they would sign up any member of their medical staff by open invitation (ostensibly to reduce the hospital's exposure under Medicare fraud and abuse statutes). In such situations, no forethought is given to the appropriate mix of panel members or to whether such members would practice quality medical care, let alone quality managed care–style medical care. In some cases, physicians join up with certain IPAs in hopes that they *won't* get any managed care business but so they can say to their colleagues that they participate in managed care.

IPAs are virtual structures for another reason. An IPA has very little tangible form. An example of the tangible form of an IPA is its "headquarters." One particular IPA of which I'm aware is physically located in the corner of a strip mall. Upon entering the office, you would see a small waiting room, the office of the administrator, the office of the finance officer, some secretarial desks and office equipment, and a souped-up personal computer that functions as the server of a local area network, perhaps tied in to offsite physicians' offices via gateways to a wide area network. Depending on its size, the IPA may also employ an information officer who manages the network, the server, and the integrity of the data used by the software run on the various terminals and hardware linkups. What you typically won't find in the IPA headquarters is an actual physician.

The group-model structure, by contrast, is quite tangible. The physicians who are part of a medical group are at risk according to the earnings of the group as a whole; in fact, the combined net income of each of the physician members of a medical group becomes the income for the group as a whole. Some groups are so large that they employ physicians who are not entitled to buy in to the ownership of the organization; some such physicians are salaried and some are contracted (with or without paying "rent," and at various levels of risk assumption), whereas others are employed on a trial basis to determine their "worthiness" to become owners. These groups have their own building in which they practice, whether the land and improvements are owned by the group or by others. For example, in North Long Beach, California, the Harriman-Jones

Medical Group (part of a physician-hospital organization with UniHealth America for some time now) occupies a very large building adjoining a major interstate, and there is no mistaking that Harriman-Jones physicians practice in this distinct location.

Group physicians are compensated according to some formula based on the net income of the group as a whole at the end of each month. If the medical group is a corporation, physicians are compensated differently according to how much and to what kind of corporate stock they own. If the medical group is a partnership, physicians are compensated either equally, according to the amount contributed to the partnership at buy-in, or according to the percentage of the group's gross or net revenues that each member generated in a given month. In either a corporate or a partnership structure, group physicians are compensated according to the financial performance of the group as a whole. If the group had an operating loss for a given month, the physician owners, like owners in any traditional business, would not get paid.

This distinction between the IPA model and the group model is very important from the standpoint of capitated managed care. In an IPA model, physician members are compensated according to how much they bill, even though the IPA as a whole might be compensated on the basis of a capitated fee with a health plan or another provider who acts as a payor. In a group model, physician members are compensated according to how well all of the physicians in the group perform good managed care medicine. For example, two physicians (one an IPA member and the other a group member) might perform a history and physical on the same patient (who might even be covered by the same health plan). The IPA physician might generate a complete battery of tests, including a stress test and a full blood panel because he or she is typically compensated according to consumption—the more billed, the more received as compensation. (Obviously, this cause–effect relationship is not absolute, especially as more IPAs are trying to cut back on wasteful practices, improve their quality, and make themselves more attractive to other payors, even though their compensation practices haven't changed accordingly and require vigilance by managers to make the organization more marketable.) The group physician, who is at risk for consumption, might take a complete history but might think twice about consuming higher-cost diagnostics like a stress test or a full blood panel, unless there is a clear medical indication that a differential diagnosis would benefit from such procedures. Some groups would authorize full blood panels on an exclusion basis, whereby the physician must justify why a full panel was consumed instead of more limited blood tests that would test for very specific blood properties. Such ratcheting of diagnostics is part of good managed care medicine and is not necessarily indicative of rationing, unless the level of managed care medicine does not improve concurrently.

Good managed care medicine, like effective capitated enrollee management, requires appropriate levels and appropriately managed information. For example, if asking very specific, fact-finding questions during the history could rule out the possibility that certain properties of blood, if tested, would have any likelihood of improving a differential diagnosis, the physician could create a more accurate diagnosis while saving the group money. In this example, by ordering tests of blood urea nitrogen (BUN) and creatinine only, the physician will generate much more cost savings than by ordering a Chem-20 (which includes BUN and creatinine among 18 other specific blood properties). All of these small diagnostic savings add up for a large group, and the monthly savings could mean the difference between a group of physicians with ownership interests receiving a paycheck and not receiving one. As someone who has helped manage a medical group that went without paychecks, I can say that this dire situation is one most managers would gladly avoid.

MSO versus PHO

Two other provider models are geared to the ever-changing relationship between managed care organization (MCO) and physician providers: management service organizations (MSOs) and physician-hospital organizations (PHOs). From the physician provider perspective, MSOs and PHOs emanate from the group-model structure and relate to market forces that are driving MCOs and larger medical groups to acquire or otherwise control physician behavior, especially when unmanaged physician behavior puts institutions at unacceptable levels of risk under capitation (see Chapter Four).

Management service organizations represent the reengineering of medical group structure to make medical groups more attractive for purchase or merger, and represent opportunities to leverage economies of scale to allow one medical group's infrastructure to manage other groups in the same marketplace. This infrastructure is either poorly defined or inherently well organized; in either case it is frequently hidden within most medical groups. The existence of this infrastructure, in whole or in

part, emanates from the nonmedical aspects of the medical group's organization, such as billing and financial counseling; finance and accounts
payable; information systems; management functions; human resources;
loss prevention services; ancillary services; clinic operations; and customer relations functions including marketing, scheduling, cashiering,
and credit/collections. The premise of MSO development is that this nonmedical infrastructure could be split off from the remainder of the medical group (e.g., physicians, their medical office building, the land value
of their medical office building, and their patient records) or sold on a
contract basis to other payors and/or providers.

In one aspect of creating an MSO, the medical group is split into two
separate legal entities (i.e., corporations), each with its own tax identification number, strategic business plan, and policies/procedures manual.
The pooled assets of the medical group's members, in conjunction with
its retained earnings (including the collection of rent from the MSO if it
continues to reside in the group's medical office building) and medical
records, and the group's land/physical plant become the assets of the
recast medical group. Its policies and procedures manuals might represent loss-prevention strategies, clinical practice parameters, malpractice
avoidance strategies, and consensus in managing medical practice under
certain contracts. Its strategic business plan may present its short- and
long-range objectives for realigning the size of the medical group, the
percentage of capitated business that it will strive to obtain/maintain, and
its strategies for managing capitated populations under my Capitated
Enrollee Management approach (see Chapter Six).

On the MSO side, the corporation obtains its own tax identification number and creates its own strategic business plan and policies/procedures manual. All of the other assets of the medical group, including the fair market
value of capital equipment and retained earnings (ancillary net income plus
administrative income via a sole-source management services agreement
with the medical group for managing the nonmedical aspects of its operations) become the asset base of a small MSO. Its employees include some
or all of the nonphysicians who were previously associated with the medical
group. Its strategic plan focuses on the MSO's ability to manage the operations of medical groups in general, including consulting income arising
from their expertise in forming other MSOs in their market area and management service income on behalf of other area medical groups. By contrast, large MSOs exist that manage specialized capitation business on a
regional or even multi-state basis on behalf of large payors and MCOs.

The reality of the formation of a small MSO by a medical group is that few such MSOs manage other medical groups, few actively solicit and receive consulting income in forming other MSOs, and many small MSOs are merely "calling cards" for would-be buyers of medical groups. The reason for the attractiveness of MSOs to MCOs, venture capital corporations, and very large medical groups is simple: The fair market value of the medical group and all of its would-be assets has been determined in advance, not at the time of sale (which would have the real potential of adding a level of goodwill above that which would reasonably be assumed to be a fair market value of any or all such assets). Since few games are played in determining a "real" value of the medical group and its medical and nonmedical assets, a purchase can be consummated relatively quickly.

If the purchaser is a PHO (see below), the purchaser may agree to purchase both the MSO and the medical group, with the purchaser agreeing to the fair market value of the MSO and the group's real estate–based assets (a process that is even easier if the MSO was recently formed) and certain prices per covered life and per noncapitated medical record. If, on the other hand, the purchaser is another medical group (ostensibly with its own MSO), only the remaining medical group would be purchased (on the basis of price per capitated life and price per noncapitated medical record), thus putting the new MSO at risk to generate other business or to get out of business.

A PHO is organized under the premise that a managed care organization (MCO) needs to control physicians, especially those medical groups that further the MCO's strategic goals, particularly in the area of controlling covered lives in a capitated marketplace. Since physician control is the MCO's valued interest, and since many MCOs are currently prohibited from owning medical practices due to restrictions such as the corporate practice of medicine, the creation of a PHO is of strategic benefit, especially to those MCOs that are nonproprietary, district-owned, or governmental organizations.

In forming a PHO, a nonprofit foundation (in some cases, a tax-exempt, public-benefit one) is created, 50 percent of which is comprised of trustees of the MCO's board and 50 percent of members of the medical group's executive board. The PHO entity (i.e., foundation) then acquires the assets of the medical group. The physicians who are part of the merged medical group are typically paid a salary by the PHO entity; when this compensation change occurs, members of the hospital who are part of the PHO entity have knowledge of physician incomes and can have a say in how the physician "employees" manage their business.

The managed care organization, or sometimes the PHO itself, might also acquire the assets of the MSO, should there be one. In such a secondary acquisition, the MCO is expanded by the addition of some or all of the former MSO employees, and the MSO assets become MCO assets. If the PHO or the MCO does not purchase the MSO, the managed care organization might choose to contract with the management services organization in managing the newly acquired medical group, either on a short-term consulting basis or as part of a longer-term contract.

Because of such interrelationships, the creation of a PHO, in part by a managed care organization, is enhanced by the medical group's preforming an MSO. While there are no guarantees that an MSO will be acquired if a PHO is formed with the remainder medical group, or that the MSO would even stay solvent if the medical group is acquired by an entity other than a PHO, MSO formation is critical in mature capitated markets. The creation of an MSO as its own entity allows for better, more prospective management of a medical group, especially when physicians are less involved in micromanagement and capital expenditure review and more involved in benefiting from the overall expertise of an organization managed by operational and financial professionals. Employees in well-run MSOs within more mature capitation markets are desirable to consultants engaged to assist in MSO formation in less mature markets, to newly formed PHOs around the country, and for professional development purposes as such employees evaluate other job opportunities in emerging MCOs, MSOs, PHOs, and medical groups.

CONTRACTING TRENDS LEADING TO CAPITATION

Capitation represents a fixed-fee, prospective payment, contractual arrangement between payors and providers. Many of the problems we've come to realize regarding the way providers deal with (or don't deal with) capitation have to do with changed priorities and strategies in managing such business. It is the lack of a willingness to change that challenges providers' responsiveness to capitation and its opportunities. For example: How did hospitals *change* with the change to DRG-based revenue?

Changes Brought About by DRGs

The surprise answer to the question just posed is that much change occurred, but only in areas that perpetuated the charade that reimbursement was continuing. As mentioned in Chapter One, the two primary areas in which change occurred with DRGs were medical records and patient accounting. In the patient accounting department (aka the business office), hybrid decision support systems were installed in the area of expected reimbursement (aka XR) computer programs, which enabled billers to maximize Medicare gross receivables and to help patient account managers predict Medicare net receivables. From the perspective of medical records, the importance of appropriate codings for Medicare patients (and especially codes that enabled hospitals to bill more to Medicare) defined a new importance of this department within the hospital. Medical records departments, prior to the installation of computerized coding software that eventually tied in to increasingly complex XR systems, were comprised of nurses and technologists who were previously untrained in the financial aspects of the hospital's operations and had to perform all medical records codings by hand.

From my perspective, the purchase and installation of computerized coding systems for hospital medical records departments represented both one of the major improvements and one of the major disappointments with regard to what was to happen later in our industry. The biggest improvement I saw was the recognition that clinical staff, originally medical records nurses and technologists, were important team members in the move toward greater hospital profitability. Subsequent trends that emerged from this event included the creation of real-time computer systems (an upgrade from large mainframes, which operated only in batch mode), the creation of PC-based local area networks that enabled diverse hospital departments to network, and the better use of previously centralized information to allow for more diffused decision making and patient care improvements. Furthermore, from this first dialogue where the medical records department was recognized as having a role in maximizing Medicare XR following the implementation of DRGs, hospital managers became less afraid to approach clinicians in other areas, especially in addressing optimal functional relationships between medical units and ancillary departments, lost charge audits, late postings of ancillary charges to bills, and current continuous quality improvement (CQI) efforts—albeit at the most preliminary stages, if in implementation at all—to redefine operations to improve both profitability and outcomes.

The most disturbing trend, however, was that hospitals resisted the opportunity to computerize their medical records at the time that infrastructure enhancement occurred with coding systems. As a result, medical records departments (in many cases, to this day) were forced to continue to maintain parallel systems: a mostly manual system of creating and updating medical records and a specialized computer system used mostly for coding purposes. While the bringing of computerization to the medical records department in the form of a multipurpose personal computer could enable medical records department heads to install spreadsheet software for budgeting, word processing software for administrative communications, and fax modems for communicating with physician offices, the sad fact is that few medical records departments have their own local area networks to allow for *concurrent* processing in all of these areas; in fact, many medical records departments have only one or two PCs (typically older models unable to take advantage of the multitasking and user-friendly interfaces so common today) that must be surrendered when a coding need arises. This reality is symptomatic of a trend that has been occurring in hospitals since original infrastructure investments in the 1980s, when personal computers were purchased for a specific application and, even today, it is that application alone that continues to limit the broader uses of such management information system (MIS) tools.

In short, what changed in hospitals with the arrival of DRGs were systems and infrastructure investment, which both strengthened profitability under Medicare and preserved a reimbursement-based methodology at a time when HCFA signaled the creation of prospective-based revenues. DRGs were viewed to be more manageable with the purchase of XR systems, whose very name suggested that reimbursement had a healthy future in the hospital industry. Infrastructure changes were also geared to making sure that more Medicare charges could be excluded from DRGs by making Medicare cost reports reflective of tremendous expansions to outpatient care and ambulatory health delivery systems; this process, part of what is known as *cost shifting,* allowed for elasticity of price for outpatient services to offset, on an incremental basis, the increasing disallowed charges on the inpatient side under DRGs. In other words, the hospital industry's strategies under DRGs were geared to (1) sheltering as many costs/charges as possible from being included under the DRG umbrella;

(2) maximizing DRG codings to squeeze as much reimbursement as possible from those cases that had to be covered by the DRG umbrella; and (3) predicting DRG deductions from revenue as far in advance as possible to give enough time to predict outliers (and, if needed and appropriate, apply for outlier payments), to predict overall deductions from revenue with enough time to find offsetting revenues to meet harsh budget expectations, and to give more opportunity for further cost shifting.

Changes That Did Not Occur with DRGs

What reactions that did not occur with the enactment of a prospective payment system related to transformational management in the wake of a marked end to reimbursement-based revenues. DRGs should have signaled the end of respiratory therapy departments, the end of phlebotomy functions within the clinical laboratory, and a concomitant reinvestment in nursing infrastructure (both pay scales and educational opportunities) to *re-include* these job functions within nursing care. Other cost-plus infrastructures that needed, and still require, reevaluation include (1) separate radiology departments and infrastructures for such services as ultrasound, nuclear medicine, tomography, MRI, lithotripsy, diagnostic radiology, and perhaps radiation therapy; (2) separate cardiovascular departments and infrastructures such as EKG, Holter, Echo, stress testing, diagnostic cardiac catheterization, angioplasty, cardiac rehab, vascular lab, and cardiovascular imaging studies; and (3) separate rehabilitation departments and infrastructures such as physical therapy, occupational therapy, speech therapy, audiology, behavioral therapy, vocational rehab and therapy, recreation therapy, music therapy, dance therapy, art therapy, and all other acute therapy services. On such unbundled, departmental levels, managers can assess such areas as service economies, profitability, and customer satisfaction as well as opportunity for outsourcing.

To date, general acute care hospitals have not yet created a wellness services department. Such a department could be comprised of proactive-based services such as education, nutritional counseling, executive fitness, weight-loss programs, smoking cessation programs, and school-based programs. These uncoordinated wellness services are often buried deep within what is now part of most hospitals' general and administrative (G&A) "department."

Other changes that need to occur involve a reexamination of the dichotomy of hospital departments between "revenue-producing" and "non-revenue-producing," which still exists even among hospitals that derive substantial revenues from capitation. The mindset that needed to occur, in reaction to PPS, is that hospital services that support other services (e.g., central supply, central sterile supply, pharmacy, and IV therapy) can no longer be considered revenue-producing. In fact, most all hospital services classified as revenue-producing are increasingly geared for a minority of a hospital's business: PPOs, private insurance, workers' compensation, and cash-paying. Compared with Medicare, these payor classes represent less than 50 percent of a hospital's business today, and even less when the current and future impacts of capitated managed care are taken into account.

Implications for Newer Contracting Trends

The implications for the changes that did not occur under DRGs involve contracting trends that were more prospective than DRGs but consistent with HCFA's original prospective payment system. Private insurance plans began to experiment with per diem payment for institutional care (a flat fee paid per day of care, either as a global, or fixed, fee for all departments or as a variable fee tied to different hospital departments) instead of discounted fee-for-service. One of the problems with per diems is that each patient needed to have a very long length of stay in order for a hospital to cover its fixed costs associated with that patient's admission. Physicians received more compensation (on a DFFS basis that continued for professional fees) the longer the patient stayed in the hospital. The countervailing force, however, was the provider review organization (PRO), which reviewed admission and discharge records on behalf of states, regional health service agencies, licensing agencies, and key payors. While per diems were, in effect, creating incentives for patients to stay in hospitals longer and to have more care covered in inpatient settings, provider review organizations became more strident in reviewing hospital admissions for appropriateness, in some cases jeopardizing certification (important to Medicare, Blue Cross, and other key payors) for hospitals that had inappropriate admissions. One of the strategies hospitals utilized to respond to PROs, while recognizing that fixed costs weren't covered on shorter lengths of stay, was to load more of the fixed cost into the first few days of care and create financial disincentives for keeping patients too long. These new per diems, called *front-loaded per diems,* involved higher per diem rates for the first few days of care and lower rates on the back end. At the same time that hospitals began to renegotiate their straight per diems for front-loaded ones, they began a long process (which continues today) to convince physicians to go along with hospitals' strategies to reduce length of stay and to practice better "managed care medicine."

Newer payor changes were also occurring. PPOs entered the scene and began providing stringent utilization review for all admissions, denying a hospital's charges where preauthorization was not obtained or where less costly alternative practices were not followed. HMOs were giving up on DFFS for expensive hospital care and instead choosing per diem—and, later, front-loaded per diem—pricing. Private insurance plans began to incorporate a case-mix indexing system, using the same indexes used by HCFA in the DRG program as multipliers against a negotiated base in the creation of indexed case rates. This methodology, still used by some Blue Shield agencies and others, is one that starts to put hospitals at risk for the care they provide. Unlike true DRG-based systems, indexed case rates make no allowances for outlier payments. Thus, hospitals that, through luck or prospective patient management (also called case management), consume fewer resources than average for a particular DRG basis, enjoy the higher case rate against the lower amount of resources consumed as incremental profit; hospitals that maintain the status quo with no infrastructure investment in prospective patient management techniques will see incremental losses per case. HMOs also started to move to global, as opposed to indexed, case rates, but only as a very temporary measure before they could more widely capitate providers to assume much larger levels of risk. The veiled lesson is that case management techniques can help a hospital achieve profitability under case rates by ensuring that hospitals spend less money than they were budgeted to spend. A prospective approach to managing patients better, both in the community as well as in the hospital, will also create a similar financial reward for hospitals under case rates. In this manner, hospitals can achieve the benefits of case rate successes without a reliance on case management.

Is Case Management the Answer?

My reader should be able to surmise that I am critical of case management as a managed care panacea. Actually, I feel that case management is useful in helping providers take a more proactive approach in patient management, but that it is only an interim step toward a new paradigm of health management. Case managers started out as good utilization review coordinators, with some experience in quality assurance. The experience of case managers is in doing retrospective studies, but the job requires real-time management. The premise of case management is to keep clinical quality high while getting managed care patients (per diem, case rate, indexed case rate, and capitation sources for revenues) discharged sooner. By lowering variable costs incrementally, more profit can be coaxed out of constrained hospital revenues. The problem is not the job of case managers but the reliance by MCO senior managers on case management as the means for better patient management. The problem, which is still compounding, involves unrealistic expectations being placed on case management as an alternative to true change.

Case management under case rates makes good sense, from the perspectives of both finance and quality. For hospitals in mature capitation markets, such as Southern California, very few MCO revenues derive anymore from case rates. Yet case management is being asked to work its magic on capitated populations, which I feel is an impossibility. Case management involves spending less; from a systems theory perspective, it improves outputs for constant or lower inputs. Under capitation, by contrast, a hospital loses money every time a capitated enrollee is admitted to a bed. Thus, a case management approach under capitation means that a hospital loses less money per capitation admission—but the hospital still always loses money. Is the value of case management to help a hospital lose less money than it would lose without case management? Is such loss minimization really a function of value? Is case management truly valuable under capitated managed care? I truly believe that case management resources are better spent in a holistic approach to enrollee wellness, and should not simply be used in a strategy to ration inpatient care and to ration longer lengths of stay.

All Roads Lead to Capitation

Capitation is the ultimate in risk-bearing payment. The opportunity for mismanaging capitation increases as providers are less prepared to manage the revenues appropriately. The missteps previously taken by the hospital industry in less risky, but equally prospective, forms of payment (see above) compromise their ability to manage capitation appropriately. In the old days, hospitals used to gauge how well they were doing by asking, "What's the census?" In comparing the census number with the total complement of beds set up and available for patients, managers could determine their vacancy rate and have a good idea of how much excess labor costs they had relative to the number of beds remaining empty. Under capitation, the reverse analysis occurs: Managers should know that their hospital loses money with each additional capitated enrollee who occupies a bed. Nowadays, "What's the census?" should be a barometer of how much money a hospital is losing, not how much it's making.

Yet the paradigm change is not widely occurring. Hospitals are seeing a greater portion of their revenues owing to capitation (if they're lucky) and are not appropriately changing to address capitation's unique situation. Case management as a patient management strategy falls noticeably short, in that hospitals which don't adopt an all-encompassing strategy for managing the health of capitated enrollees will make no money under capitation, whether or not they have invested in case management. Case management will measure only how much money such hospitals lose from their capitated business and how much money hospitals with a dwindling amount of case rates will retain as income.

Hospitals' ability to get "lean and mean" under capitation is compromised by the myriad departments and infrastructures that remain unconsolidated (and exist only because Medicare *used to* reimburse costs, and because such costs *used to* be done on a cost-plus basis). As suggested earlier, hospitals are so far behind on changing to prospective payment that the funds to subsidize their change will go away as more of their business becomes capitated; such changes include eliminating the obsolete structures they continue to maintain (e.g., respiratory therapy and phlebotomy), and by the delay in developing infrastructures for enhancing and managing wellness. In addition, the anachronistic, single-use computer systems that exist in key hospital departments will jeopardize hospitals' ability to respond to opportunities created by capitation without substantial, all-at-once capital infusions that should have been made all along.

Capitation is also highly desirable for HMOs. As Chapter Three will show, HMOs make lots of money from commercial capitation, and even more from Medicare Risk capitation. HMOs have discovered that if hospitals are ready to bear risk in the form of case rates, then they are certainly ready for capitation, to the extent providers are buying and to the extent HMOs are selling. Capitation is tempting for providers, especially medical groups willing to accept full-risk medical capitation; large capitation checks, sometimes in six or seven figures, paid religiously every month to providers as a 1990s form of PIP, are very hard to resist. Capitation is also a strategy that the HMO industry in mature markets has been pushing for the last five years, and it is the current strategy for emerging capitation markets around the country. Capitation represents a way for HMOs to get out of the healthcare delivery business.

WHAT PROVIDERS NEED TO KNOW ABOUT THE INSURANCE BUSINESS

An important lesson providers must learn about the insurance business concerns underwriting. Underwriting represents the process of selecting, classifying, evaluating, and assuming risks according to their insurability. According to the underwriting process, the insurance company determines how much liability it can insure against; and the actuarial process, using actuarial mathematics, determines at what premium level such insurability can be offered to customers.

Another important lesson providers must learn about the insurance business concerns how much insurability the underwriting process allows. Let's say that the underwriting process suggests that an insurance company can offer $500,000 worth of coverage and that the actuarial process determines that $5,000 worth of premium is required for this level of coverage. If the insurance company charges $5,000 in premium for such insurance coverage, the upper limit of the coverage for that premium— $500,000—is known as the *stop-loss limit;* in other words, the insurance company can offer coverage only to the stop-loss limit of $500,000. The reverse scenario, common in capitation, is also true: An insurance company can offer a provider $5,000 in capitation payment (assuming the insurer is operating on a break-even basis with no contribution to overhead or profit—a highly unlikely scenario for any business, even a nonproprietary one) to cover $500,000 of liability. The important point is that it is the *insurer* who is doing the actuarial math and the underwriting analysis, not the provider; the provider is blind to the processes used to determine the pricing offered. In this example, the payor may offer the provider $2,500 capitation for a stop-loss limit of $500,000, representing a potential 50% profit margin of which the provider is unaware.

Coverage required above a stop-loss level involves "reinsurance," since it involves a level of risk not included in the original underwriting process. Reinsurance is an insurance product, more expensive than standard insurance, that covers claims made above stop-loss levels; by definition, such coverage involves only those cases with the highest risk and the most significant losses. To keep reinsurance rates lower, insurance companies try to keep stop-loss levels as high as possible. Hence, insurers will more actively seek providers willing to accept higher stop-loss levels; in competition for coverage or capitation, such providers willing to accept risk will have a selection advantage over more risk-averse providers looking for safer (lower) stop-loss levels. From a provider perspective, physicians looking to negotiate for capitated rates want to get the best (highest) price for the safest (lowest) stop-loss requirements—but only up to a point: Providers asking capitators for below-market stop-loss levels could convey a shakiness of operation or a lack of capacity to accept high levels of risk. On the other hand, capitators might think twice about a small-sized provider looking for stop-loss levels at, say, $1 to $2 million, because of the fair likelihood that such an enterprise will lack the systems and capabilities to manage risk appropriately and will fail quickly, thus requiring the capitator to resell a population in the same market to the same providers. The expectation here is that the capitator will have to offer concessions (like below-market stop-loss levels and/or above-market capitation rates) to resell risk that wouldn't be necessary the first time the business is offered to providers.

Capitation is an insurance product, not a healthcare product. The HMOs that offer capitation are really health insurance companies. Like HMOs offered as options of traditional insurance companies (like Aetna, Cigna, Prudential, and Traveler's), stand-alone health maintenance organizations (like PacifiCare, FHP, Foundation Health, U.S. Healthcare, QualMed, HealthNet [now part of Wellpoint], and Maxicare, to name but just a few) are regulated by state insurance and/or corporation agencies, are insured by underwriters, offer premiums that are based on actuarial projections, and are typically managed by insurance industry executives. The owners and managers of HMOs owe their allegiance to the insurance industry and not to the healthcare industry.

Where HMOs' allegiances lie is of substantial importance to providers. Members of the healthcare industry, unlike members of the insurance industry, are of very hardy stock. The healthcare industry has historically approached adversity and adverse financial realities, and found a way to make them work. When Medicare instituted DRG-based payment as part of its prospective payment system in 1983, thereby doing away with cost-plus reimbursements and hospitals' beloved PIPs, providers found a way to make prospective payment work. For better or worse, they instituted changes in their charging and coding practices to make DRGs as profitable as possible. In other words, providers didn't lament that their costs would rise and that their profits would fall but found ways to realign their infrastructure to make the most profits possible out of DRGs.

When HCFA instituted the resource-based relative value scale (RBRVS) in 1993 to bring medical practice more in line with a prospective payment system, of course providers lamented. However, their lamenting turned into proactive strategizing, and charging systems have been revised to maximize RBRVS payment while practice guidelines have changed to better align clinical practice with standardized RBRVS rates. Finally, many large, quality providers are trying to make a go with capitation. There are software packages on the market to receive capitation payments and provide for simplified payment of subcapitation to other providers and vendors, including the use of electronic data interchange (EDI) to make the management process paperless. Providers are also hiring consultants and spending money on professional education to learn more about capitation and the impact it will have on their businesses. In short, the healthcare industry's history is in fighting back in the face of change and potential financial adversity. As you will see in the next chapter, the insurance industry's history is in running away from adversity.

Chapter Three

The Transformation of the Healthcare Market to Capitation

This chapter will show how capitation emerged within the healthcare marketplace, the nature of the long-range positioning of the HMO industry in introducing capitation to an unsuspecting provider public, and how the marketplace is being transformed as a result. The illustration on the next page will assist the reader in grasping this transformation.

UNDERSTANDING THE FINANCIAL NATURE OF HMOs

HMOs are commonly viewed by the public as companies (such as FHP, Inc.; Pacificare Health Systems, Inc.; Cigna Healthplans, Inc.). To the extent that there is advertising, the public might also view HMOs as product offerings—such as the "Secure Horizons" Medicare Risk product of Pacificare, the "FHP Senior" Medicare Risk product of FHP, and the "CareAmerica 65+" Medicare Risk product of UniHealth America–owned CareAmerica Health Plans. The public might readily perceive that the offering of HMO-structured coverage also allows traditional insurance companies to broaden their portfolio of the health insurance products they sell, which has traditionally helped insurance companies position themselves to their customers: large employers; unions; and third-party administrators on behalf of smaller unions, benefit trusts, ERISA plans, and employers. The offering of HMO coverage is the common vehicle by which insurance companies promote that they have "triple option" coverage for customers seeking health insurance. For many years, the offering of "dual option" coverage (private indemnity or

A Schematic History of Managed Care and Capitation in Southern California

HMO Delivery System—1980s through 1991

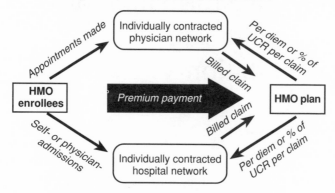

HMO Delivery System—1991 through 1993

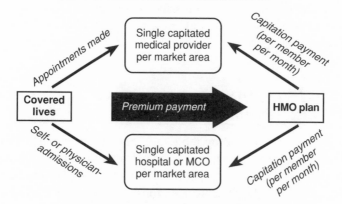

HMO Delivery System—Newest Paradigm

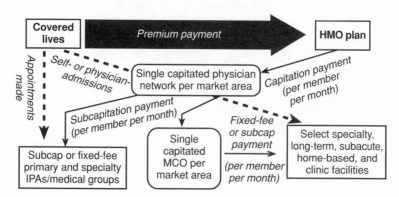

Source: © David Samuels & Associates, 1994.

group insurance coupled with PPO-structured coverage) has usually been sufficient in distinguishing these insurance companies from firms selling only "traditional" health insurance.

Traditional health insurance is a euphemism for group insurance or private indemnity insurance, which pays providers on a gross percentage of charges (typically "80/20," whereby the plan pays 80 percent with the remaining 20 percent charged to the insured as a co-payment) or on a discounted fee-for-service (DFFS) basis (whereby a dollar limitation is applied instead of a UCR, against which the 80/20 is applied; disallowed fees or fees that exceed the dollar cap are also charged to the insured as an additional share of cost). Providers receive the most money for services rendered with traditional insurance, and they tend to jump through any hoops the insurance company may impose in order to retain this business.

On this note, many providers still bill traditional health insurance companies as a courtesy and convenience to their patients because of the relative "creaminess" of this business compared with PPO and capitated HMO business that may also be held by the provider. The hoops for the traditional health insurance business may also include what I call claims department shenanigans, which might include lost claims, claims adjudicated against the wrong insured, unexplained processing delays (which may be entirely legitimate but are not freely communicated to the provider or the provider's billing agent except when questioned and with the level of detail commensurate with "need to know"), and various bureaucratic procedures. The point is that providers put up with these peccadilloes; they hire additional billers or collectors as necessary, and they make do with reduced cash flow and increased deductions from revenue.

The PPO-structured health insurance is less creamy than group insurance but still relatively profitable on a level of service basis compared with capitated HMO business. Under the PPO structure, the insurance company sought to insulate itself from some risks by beginning to control provider behavior and by beginning to control the behavior of insureds who consume services by creating financial incentives and disincentives. In the PPO arrangement, "preferred panels" of providers were established as a means of cutting the sheer volume of claims that the insurance company had to process and adjudicate each day. The panels also created contractual norms for providers, who had to agree to dollar thresholds for specific procedures billed, against which a percentage of charges would apply. The quid pro quo for the providers who joined the panel became a raising of reimbursement levels from the traditional 80 percent to a more palatable 90 percent of charges. (Of course, providers not on the panels would be paid "something," but more typically at the 35 to 50 percent level.) The preferred providers also learned that PPOs were not risk assumptive, in that charges either disallowed by the insurance company or in excess of the dollar caps were largely chargeable to the patient or to the patient's guarantor as additional shares of cost, or to traditional insurances that were secondarily billed to the patient or guarantor.

The motivation of insurance companies to offer PPO offerings was purely one of profit, although the profit was seen—sometimes—only by providers. What customers saw was the marketing hype claiming that the cost of coverage was lower for the employer (which sometimes meant that the employee shared in this cost savings on the basis of premium paid); that providers were specially selected by the plan (with obvious connotations of enhanced quality, even though there was never any meat to the quality claims offered by insurance companies when dealing with PPOs—quality was not measured or assured on a real-time basis, and for that matter was even poorly defined); and that there was utilization review.

From a profit-oriented perspective, managed care without capitation represents cost inefficiencies and requires tremendous infrastructures. This reality, in conjunction with the need to outsource the management of healthcare for HMO populations in a growing number of markets around the country, is why capitation is becoming a valuable commodity for health industry providers. Yet providers should recognize the old adage "caveat emptor." The buyer must be very aware.

WHICH INDUSTRY?

As discussed in Chapter Two, the HMO industry is more reflective of the insurance industry than of the healthcare industry. The leaders of HMOs, with the exception of HSI chief executive officer Dr. Malik Hassan and a handful of others, generally come from the insurance industry. The insurance industry's value system is one of avoiding rather than overcoming substantial losses. The healthcare industry's value system is associated with finding ways to make profits from adverse situations, even if the odds are stacked against it, as is often the case in the early days of capitation. The insurance industry backbone of HMOs does not share this value system.

In fact, the insurance industry backbone of HMOs in general is very risk averse. If costs and claims are higher than budgeted, and only if the losses are fairly minimal, insurance companies will first try to raise rates. If rates can't be raised high enough to overcome adverse claims experiences, insurance companies will then get out of the business. Doubters need look only at the number of insurance companies still providing earthquake coverage in California, hurricane insurance in Florida, automobile insurance in New York and other states with high loss ratios (percentage of losses incurred against premiums collected), directors and officers liability insurance in states without tort reform, and medical malpractice insurance just about anywhere. When costs are higher than budgeted, insurance companies stop writing new policies and drop coverages in order to get out of "unprofitable" markets. This history is the exact opposite of the healthcare industry's experience.

Capitation recognizes that health plans are not adept at managing care. They are uncomfortable with the huge infrastructures they must maintain to collect billed claims, adjudicate them, pay them, and defend against provider challenges of denied claims. The HMOs have been out of place in hiring good people with health insurance backgrounds to process and adjudicate claims, and have been unsuccessful in using non-healthcare insurance industry management principles and productivity standards (such as working with claims adjusters) in managing claims personnel within provider organizations (e.g., a physician's front office personnel). The infrastructure required to manage such unfamiliar processes is expensive and foreign to traditional insurance industry practices. The primary attractiveness of capitation to HMOs is the fact that it represents outsourcing; its profitable nature is secondary.

Capitation is the means by which payors outsource their healthcare insurance products. *Outsourcing* means that the responsibility for performing a certain function is sold to someone else for a relatively fixed fee; in return, the outsourcing entity can still collect fees for a service that is performed by others. HMOs still collect premiums when capitation is paid (for groups of providers to manage books of business for which the management responsibility has been sold by the HMOs), and providers paid capitation have the contractual responsibility for managing specific, capitated enrollees.

Capitation represents the means by which the insurance industry roots of HMOs can do what they know how to do: sell premium. HMOs are demonstrating their skill at (1) creating advertising campaigns to sell more premium, (2) defeating or lobbying against legislation that would jeopardize their ability to sell more premium, (3) creating specific promotions during periods of "open enrollment" to compete with other HMOs and other insurance products to sell more premium, and (4) investing in health- and wellness-enhancing causes and foundations to improve their image—and to sell more premium. Premium sales are the lifeblood of the insurance industry, and the HMO industry is no exception. Capitated providers need to realize that such advertising and such increases in new premiums to HMOs do not accrue to their capitated arrangements; instead, the incremental profits are used to fund other capitation deals.

As incremental HMO enrollees are managed through incremental or expanded capitation arrangements, the health plans can sell more premium without having to manage those enrollees. The cycle continues as HMOs sell more premium until a critical mass is reached, whereby the HMO can apply to HCFA for a permit to sell Medicare Risk premium to seniors and other Medicare-eligible populations. Since Medicare Risk premium is substantially more profitable than commercial risk, the impetus to create capitated arrangements for Medicare populations is all the more enticing. And as more enrollees can be managed within increasing capitation arrangements, the HMOs can sell even more premium: both commercial and Medicare Risk premium.

PROBLEMS WITH TRADITIONAL MANAGED CARE

The key problem with traditional managed care is that there are no standards. There are no standard definitions, no standards in terms of what customers should be entitled to receive, and no standards in terms of the roles of physicians and hospitals in caring for customers, all the more so for common customers. Without standards, customers have no new expectations for managed care other than their perceptions of how managed care needs to change to accommodate previous expectations of quality. Quality is not defined, quality is not managed on a real-time basis, and the imperatives for managing quality—whatever it is—are higher for inpatient than outpatient care. Finally, one of the biggest problems with traditional managed care is the fixation on relationships between payors and providers, with no attention paid to consumers.

Consumerism is the missing element in traditional managed care, whether capitated or noncapitated. Capitation is hidden from consumers, consumers are excluded from decision making among providers and payors, and consumers are treated as malleable nonentities. In traditional managed care, consumers are account numbers, social security numbers, and claims opportunities. To be sure, in traditional forms of capitated managed care, payors treat capitated providers as consumers and capitated enrollees are considered to be "commodities" sold to the lowest bidder. More than a few things are inherently wrong with this attitude.

First and foremost, healthcare consumers are dynamic human beings, capable of change. They are capable of transformational change, if providers can recognize two truths: (1) consumers do not enjoy being dependent on providers and (2) they want control of their own lives. The attitude that consumers are dependent on providers for all health information is a 1970s attitude, developed long before the computerization of our society and the popularization of the Internet and proprietary, online services. In some cases, consumers have access to more and better health information than their providers do. Consumers want and deserve proactive guidance from their physicians and caregivers so that they can lead healthier lives and reduce (or eliminate) their dependence on providers. This phenomenon has not yet hit the HMO industry as a whole, except for some staff-model HMOs.

Capitated enrollees should be considered more of a potential community of members than a herd of cattle. While populations of capitated enrollees are grouped geographically for sale to providers by payors, the populations themselves are hard to organize and manage as a group because their locations are discontiguous within a geographic region. Nevertheless, the sense of community is a human need, one long ignored by the healthcare industry under traditional managed care. In his fascinating book *Parzival's Briefcase: Six Practices and a New Philosophy for Healthy Organizational Change* (San Francisco: Chronicle Books, 1993), Tony Smith, PhD, noted the following:

> We have a need to know one another, to serve one another, and to be part of something larger than ourselves. Members of a healthy community are awake to their interests and those of the organization. Not ruled by expediency or fear, these people are free to be unique and are able to share moral bonds and limits; they are interested in obedience to contribute and able to move beyond an obsession with their rights. (page 198)

People in organized groups want to evolve into self-fulfilling and mutually supportive communities. The ideal suggested by Dr. Smith is entirely possible and attainable within capitated managed care (and is

discussed in greater detail in Chapter Six). The elemental change is to
recognize that capitated enrollees want, and need, to change; with capitated enrollees on the same team, and with a desire to improve—and perhaps, at some point, take responsibility for—their own health status,
transformational changes in how capitated managed care can occur could
result in a positive-sum ("win–win") game for payors and providers. The
failings of traditional managed care in helping consumers to change and
to improve themselves could not logically occur as long as such changes
negatively impact providers under such a continued system (e.g., reductions in customer consumption negatively affect providers who are compensated on the basis of consumption).

HOW TRADITIONAL MANAGED CARE
IS SOLD TO CONSUMERS

Managed care plan enrollees need to be transformed into intelligent pur-
chasers who are told how capitation works, how they can help make managed care succeed in ways that do not require them to be waiting in physicians' offices or cooped up in hospital beds, and how they can gain control
of their lives—all the while helping providers to save money. Providers
need to be assured that investing in their enrollees will help them manage
their own constrained resources while improving the quality and healthiness of enrollees' lives—in effect, transforming their perspective from con-
trollers (a role everybody hates) to enablers (a less hated role, and perhaps
a respected one). This change in perspective will represent a tremendous
shift from how HMOs are now positioned in the marketplace.

How HMOs Sell in the General Marketplace

HMOs cannot yet boast about transformations in consumer behavior related to their lifestyles or in provider behavior related to helping enrollees (not just patients) lead their own lives, armed with the intelligence
to make appropriate health purchases and make well-intentioned lifestyle
choices. Instead, HMOs are caught in their current strategy of selling
premium, getting employers to buy capitated products, getting physicians
to join capitation-based medical groups, discouraging all but the best
managed care physicians to continue practicing in IPAs, and selling more
premium in general. We see how HMOs sell to employers and providers
in the general marketplace. Yet, how do they sell to the general public?

How HMOs Are Sold to the Public

Since the public has not yet been transformed into knowledgeable health-care consumers, their view of HMOs is about as narrow as their view of hospitals. Just as a "good" hospital is often measured by the temperature of the food it serves and the cleanliness of the lobby (which the patient rarely sees), an HMO is judged as good according to the nationality of the physicians contracted with it, the hospitals advertised as "affiliated" with it, and how much it costs. There are quality elements in these measures, but the level of sophistication about quality and the extent to which it is present are quite basic.

Hospitals have been promoting themselves to the public on the basis of quality for the last 25 years, even though the hospital industry has not attempted to standardize the definition of quality for 20 of those years and still lacks a gold standard. The old phrase "Beauty is in the eye of the beholder" applies to quality as well, since individuals set their own specifications of what quality is and when quality has been achieved. Rather than take a lead from traditional business in asking random samples of consumers to help measure quality as it is perceived—through sophisticated phone, mail, and in-person sampling techniques, including expensive focus groups—the healthcare industry has wrongly chosen to ignore reality and instead capitalize on consumers' lack of knowledge about the industry by promoting everything as high quality.

Quality, Quality, Quality

> Come to Community Medical Center—we've got quality facilities, quality physicians, quality nurses, quality chefs, and a long-standing reputation for quality. Heck, we're bursting with quality. Come to Community Medical Center, the quality hospital practicing quality medicine in a quality manner to a quality-conscious community. You want quality? We've got the highest quality!

The tactic of selling healthcare on the basis of quality worked during the 1970s and early 1980s because the notion of quality went unchallenged by consumers. Besides, the term *quality* was used so much that consumers just assumed it was always there. It wasn't until the late 1980s, when the state of Pennsylvania began releasing Medicare mortality statistics by DRGs for its hospitals to news media that consumer groups started a national inquiry into how good providers are at treating the sick. About that same time, we saw an increase in consumerism and in public interest groups that have been following the practices of the health insurance industry, hospitals, and especially physicians. Different state governments, such as that of Florida, started making medical malpractice claims and medical quality assurance records available to others, including putting hospitals at risk for the quality of their physicians (measured in settled or adjudicated malpractice and/or medical quality assurance claims). Quality was still poorly perceived by the public (food, cleanliness, and price), but the mystique was starting to erode.

In the late 1980s, the Joint Commission on Accreditation of Healthcare Organizations (JCAHO) indicated that hospitals without a means of collecting and measuring clinical outcomes data (including disease staging by DRG, a methodology by which morbidity and mortality data by DRG are stratified according to the severity of the condition; for example, were 30 annual deaths from pneumonia associated with the simplest forms of pneumonia or the most severe form?) would not receive accreditation, which has implications for the ability of such hospitals to treat people under Medicare, Medicaid, Workers Compensation, and most private insurance plans (including their HMO products). All of a sudden, hospitals and MCOs began doing disease staging and attempting to create rather crude outcomes statistics (crude in that there was generally no multiyear trending being done because the efforts were so new). The hospital industry is still in the midst of "backfilling" and of praying to any god that will listen that the empirical data will support their long-standing public pronouncements about having the highest levels of quality.

While private-sector hospitals were using the Q word like used-car salespersons, some public-sector agencies started to test the level of quality they provided. In the early 1980s, the County of Los Angeles's Department of Health Services, for example, instituted a quality measurement and improvement program called the Patient Services Improvement Program (PSIP, later changed to Health Services Improvement Program, or HSIP), which, over approximately a 10-year period, attempted to measure and reduce patient waiting times in clinics and emergency departments, increase the number of patients who received all needed services in a timely manner (improved service coordination), measure and improve Medicaid enrollees' satisfaction with the level and manner of services provided, and improve the image that county facilities and divisions had of themselves. These process improvements were initiated with external consultants knowledgeable about the work of W. Edwards Deming and the evolving field of continuous quality improvement (CQI), with later implementation, education, and facilitation occurring internally. With LA County's PSIP-related activities, and various similar programs in the public sector occurring in the mid-1980s, quality was measured in the public sector long before the private sector came up with operational definitions or began its own fact-finding. The private sector took the easy way out by taking its public rhetoric at face value.

The problem with this belated fact-finding, though, is that any outcomes results that hospitals have discovered, or are now turning up, are being viewed as great discoveries that JCAHO would want to see. The spirit of JCAHO's outcomes requirement is not that providers should have outcomes reports to hold up to the surveyor team, but that outcomes are really tools for higher-level results reporting. *Outcomes are not the ends; they are the means.* The toughest challenge to outcomes management is also the most odious: having to use outcomes results as a tool to change provider behavior. For example, does a hospital's knowing that 65 percent of all deliveries are by C-section make a difference to anybody, except for a reporter looking for a juicy story?

A 65 percent C-section rate is clearly suboptimal, for it indicates that obstetricians (and, to a much lesser extent, family physicians) are probably rushing to do repeat Caesareans on all women (at much higher cost with no clear relationship to medical need or physician habit) instead of just those who attempted vaginal birth after Caesarean (VBAC) and were unsuccessful or women of such risk status that VBAC would be medically inadvisable. The real challenge for hospitals is to use the statistic as a means of changing obstetricians' behavior and practice techniques so that subsequent reports will show fewer C-sections being performed.

Another use of outcomes statistics as a tool for change is even tougher. A hospital finds that 25 percent of simple pneumonia admissions resulted in death, for example. The data also are able to stratify those deaths according to the physician actually treating the patients. How does a hospital use data that might show that certain physicians treating patients of similar risk status—but an expectation that there would be very few deaths, given that it is "simple" pneumonia—have more incidents of death than all of the other physicians practicing at the hospital? The hospital's reaction could easily be clouded if those physicians are more loyal to the hospital than others, give better business, and/or volunteer their time on various committees and in community service activities. In short, the tough issue is how hospitals should be managing the data they are now collecting, especially if the data show that the hospitals are of considerably less quality than is told to the public. Or, put another way, should hospitals ask the right questions even if they're afraid of the wrong answers?

HMOs started out promoting on the basis of quality according to the stated quality of the members of their network, most notably hospitals. One of the reasons HMOs couldn't get as much promotion mileage from the quality of their physician network was that in many states physicians were prohibited from advertising, which is still the case in a minority of states. Even among physicians who advertise their quality, it is done in a very low-key manner with no data available to substantiate any claim of quality on the basis of outcomes— hence, no such claim is ever made. In all, claims of having high quality make for good ad copy. "All our physicians are board certified" is a popular claim that has an unclear relationship to outcomes or to whether better care will be rendered. Board certification is also an elusive measure for gauging whether a physician practices good "managed care medicine."

No one seems to be teaching the art of managed care medicine in addition to the art of medicine. There is a huge difference. Board certification seems to be an appropriate gauge to ensure that the "art of medicine" is practiced appropriately by physicians. In this sense, there may be some link to quality. Who, however, trains physicians how to diagnose without the luxury of ordering every test possible? How do physicians learn the art of ordering very specific lab tests (rather than complete panels) based on a patient's history and symptomatology alone? From what source do physicians learn which very specific questions should be asked to generate a 5-minute history that is as revealing as a complete 30-minute history? How do physicians learn to gather more, and more specific, information from a shortened physical examination with a high degree of touch instead of conducting complete one-hour physicals? In short, from what source do physicians learn how to maximize outputs while minimizing inputs? This new perspective is its own art form, and is not generally taught in medical school, internships, or internal or family medicine residency rotations. This art is not measured, let alone covered, on medical board examinations. Therefore, what is board certification really measuring or monitoring in the world of capitated managed care?

How HMOs Are Sold to Employers and Unions

HMOs are sold to employers and unions primarily on the bases of employer cost, employee cost, and employee health. Their primary sales vehicle is an HMO plan that is priced competitively with other employer health products (e.g., HMO, PPO, and AHP) in the market. The HMO account managers offer different plans and sales strategies for different sized employers, with the best features and lowest prices offered to the biggest employers willing to lock in for extended periods. As discussed in Chapter Two, the HMOs also sell EPO products to channel uncommitted employers to the "HMO side" more gradually, but typically within a year of first contact. And since most employer benefit trusts and unions negotiate directly with third-party administrators (TPAs, who generally must hold a broker's license to sell premium to their clients), the HMO has its own positioning strategy to get TPAs to sign up their clients to its health plans.

Most HMO account executives, like good salespeople, promise more to employers than is typically delivered. While every HMO positions its products on the basis of price (both cost to employer and cost to employee), there's very little differentiation, since there is, or eventually will be, market parity on the basis of HMO price. One competitor may slice a percent or two off the price, which others may match. Even in mature capitation markets in the mid-1990s, we are not yet witnessing more than a few HMOs differentiating on anything but price. Capitation provides a pricing methodology that enables HMOs to compete for premium dollar on price, because its expenses are relatively fixed (see Chapter Four). In immature capitation markets, HMOs sell their products to employers on the bases of employee health (measured by fewer sick days and improved physical conditioning), less paid time off (ostensibly for fewer visits to providers, especially those who ration), reduced employee turnover, and higher employee morale. Research from the early 1990s has shown that there are no empirical data to support these sales claims; in fact, the research shows that there are no measurable differences in morale, employee health, absenteeism, and turnover among all forms of health insurance, whether group insurance, HMO, or PPO. With very similar pricing among the three at the time, a new differentiation strategy was the obvious next step for attracting HMO market share.

Employers reacted negatively to these early reports that HMOs were providing no differentiated product while they were charging group insurance–type rates for similar results. HMOs in the late 1980s and early 1990s were looking for outsourcing methods to reduce their operating costs so that they could offer lower-priced premium to the most profitable potential customers. Capitation emerged as the perfect discounting vehicle for HMOs, because it allowed them to be more aggressive in discounting premium than competing PPO, AHP, and group insurance products providing essentially DFFS-based pricing. The timing was also excellent, considering the multiyear recession of the late 1980s and early 1990s and the receptivity of employers and unions to concessions on premium pricing. The same timing that saw widespread capitation in mature markets (50 percent or higher HMO penetration) like Southern California (Los Angeles, Orange, and San Diego counties); Minneapolis/St. Paul, Minnesota; and Worcester, Massachusetts, is now proving its value in more immature markets (such as the Southeast, Mid-Atlantic, and Midwestern regions of the United States): The economy is still fragile, imminent healthcare reform has died, and what little indemnity insurance that remains is priced so high that employers can no longer afford the luxury of "unmanaged" care.

How HMOs Are Sold to Middlemen

The old style of premium sales was to create a sales force of brokers to sell premium, paid entirely on a commission basis. The high commission rates were promised to brokers based on the availability of high premium prices to absorb this variable expense. Since brokers' licenses in most states are attainable by a relatively straightforward examination process, insurance companies were never really short of brokers willing to sell premium. Some insurance companies, like Prudential, employ brokers who sell only Prudential products; others are members of the American Independent Agents Association, and sell a variety of insurance products and health insurance plans through the same agent structure. Finally, there are also agents who sell Blue Cross and Blue Shield health insurance products based on the premise that both insurance companies coordinate their products and services. While this coordination continues in some states and regions, there are others, such as California, where the two agencies compete. To be sure, the recent rebuff in April 1995 by Wellpoint Healthcare (formerly a wholly owned subsidiary of Blue Cross of California, which has since merged with HSI) of an acquisition offer by Blue Shield of California, is indicative of the fierce rivalry that exists between these former cooperative health insurance companies. Yet even in California, most Blue Cross brokers can also sell Blue Shield plans. The insurance industry is bracing for a vituperative testing of this long-standing "partnership" in contracting with shared brokers.

It is likely that the broker structure in selling premiums may be breaking down, given that premium competition has cut back on the availability of commissions anywhere near what brokers are accustomed to receiving. This cutting back of premiums and—sooner rather than later—attractive commission rates will result in a transformation of how insurance companies sell premium. For example, are brokers still needed if health insurance companies and HMOs cut back to the level of employing their own internal sales force? What are the implications for the broker/independent agent structures if HMOs outsource premium marketing to ad agencies willing to accept vendor capitation (see Chapter Seven) or subcapitated sales marketing to ASOs (independent or part of MSOs) willing to accept incrementally higher subcapitation rates to bear the HMO's risk for hitting sales targets?

The use of TPAs in the marketplace is also changing. TPAs, by virtue of their broker's licenses, are valuable commodities in mature capitation markets, regardless of the scope and size of their client base. For example, MCOs interested in competing with HMOs (currently a death wish, but the market is becoming so fierce that anything is possible) on a direct contracting basis can, theoretically, buy a TPA not for its clients but for its license. The MCO, through the TPA structure, can create a competing benefit plan to sell to employers, perhaps including an undercutting of parity-level premium in that market. If the MCO, through the TPA, can assure the employer of appropriate depth and breadth of coverage for that particular market, it has the opportunity of stealing market share from the payors doing business in that market.

Large, self-funded benefit trusts (like the California Public Employees Retirement System, CAL-PERS) have been able to use size and volume as leverage to negotiate the lowest healthcare premium prices nationwide, in many cases "below retail." CAL-PERS's achievements in obtaining these low rates occurred without a TPA. The trend by unions to continue to pay TPAs for shopping for rates and for claims management is being challenged, especially as TPAs are seeing competition from ASOs willing to provide similar services at less cost.

WHAT FALLS THROUGH THE CRACKS IN THE CAPITATION TRANSFORMATION

It is my belief that much of the mess the current healthcare delivery system is in results from poor levels of information and a pattern of misinformation. To this day, the news media, which are eager to cover stories related to healthcare reform, medical and hospital quality, and the effects of capitation, receive misinformation and partial knowledge. For example, many news media personnel still believe that capitation is a form of reimbursement and that it is a flat monthly fee paid for each patient. This payment mechanism, described in this manner, is called a *case price*. Capitation, as you should know by now, involves a payment for a member of an HMO's plan for whom capitated risk is being sold. The confusion exists because there are certain elements about capitated managed care that HMOs either don't tell or tell only partially. As we'll see, the existence of capitation—and what that means—is one of those certain trade secrets.

Choice

HMOs typically sell to employers on the basis of the huge amount of choices that employees and their dependents could have: choice of gatekeeper, choice of hospital, and—in certain self-referral option (whereby certain enrollees deemed attractive to the HMO—like Medicare Risk—can choose specialists themselves rather than rely upon their gatekeepers' choices) and POS plans—choice of specialist. HMOs provide guidebooks to these consumers to perpetuate this illusion: providers' names, board certifications, hours of operation, languages spoken, and sometimes even the name of their medical school. Employees are given a period of time to select a gatekeeper, sometimes in conjunction with hospitals and MCOs at which these gatekeepers practice. With sophisticated information management systems, including the Internet, proprietary online services, and regional bulletin board services (BBSs), consumers have access to tremendous amounts of information about these providers, not to mention word-of-mouth endorsements from family, friends, and neighbors. Many consumers will call the physicians' offices, talk to office staff, tour the offices and clinics, and tour the hospital during this period. Through whatever process taken, consumers are given access to selection information, and in the time allotted to them they are generally vigilant in making what they feel is the most informed choice of hospital provider and primary care physician to serve as gatekeeper. On the surface, it would appear that consumers have made an informed choice of health plan provider.

The stability of such a choice, and the legitimacy of the process used by consumers to arrive at that choice, is vastly different from reality by virtue of the existence of subcapitation. As mentioned earlier, subcapitation involves the reparceling of risk by capitated providers to other providers. In the future, and with data to support the decision making, subcapitation will be made more often on the basis of outcomes and incremental value. In the present tense, however, most all subcapitation is contracted on the basis of price alone. In this way, most providers sell primary care risk to a primary care group willing to accept maximum risk (both volume and high stop loss) for the lowest subcapitation rate. Such providers may, to the extent they can, negotiate with panels and groups of specialists to assume maximum specialty risk for the lowest subcapitation rate. This practice undermines the integrity of commercial capitation and the appropriateness of capitation and subcapitation rates—new paradigms which are discussed in Chapter Six.

The bottom line, however, is that consumers are not told something very important. Consumers are not told that subcapitation means that they have no real choice of the providers they see. No matter how exacting the selection process, the ultimate choice of primary and specialty providers aligned to capitated enrollee populations will be decided by representatives of professional service organizations motivated almost solely on price. The illusion is continued when enrollees seek care from the providers *they* chose.

Rather than acknowledging that responsibility for a member's care was resold to another provider (whom the member did not choose), the chosen provider's staff, if pressed, might come up with an excuse (a lie) for why the member must see the other provider. Maybe the member is told that the physician group is closed to new appointments for six months, or that an appointment can't be scheduled anytime soon because of volume, short-staffedness, and so on; instead, the member might be told that he or she is authorized to go to another specific provider group, perhaps more convenient to the member, which has more immediate appointment availability. The member typically will not be told that it is this other provider group that has accepted the liability (and the subcapitation) for his or her care, and the care for his or her family as well. Changes in hospital provider, created when capitated MCOs subcapitate to other institutions, are also not divulged to members as being a function of subcapitation arrangements. The HMOs usually inform consumers that they might not be able to see the providers they choose, but usually don't disclose the reason (like subcapitation) that the reassignment occurs.

The particularly troubling part of the illusion of choice is how important members hold provider choice in selecting one HMO over another and how some health plans so overuse the concept of choice that it sounds like hospitals' overuse of the word *quality*. There are HMOs and HMO product names that use the word *choice,* there are plans that use themes related to choice heavily in their promotional and media campaigns, and HMOs that create high-class print media and brochure copy that emphasize the extent to which consumers have substantial choice in the physicians and hospitals they can select.

This element of choice is a fact of life about capitation and not a pattern of deceptive business practices used by HMOs. To be sure, most all HMOs are absolved of legal responsibility for patient management when the capitation contract is signed. The HMO believes, in good faith, that the elements of choice will be preserved by providers receiving capitation for their health maintenance. Yet the HMO allows providers to subcapitate in extending additional program flexibility, economies of scale, and better member choice, and additional value to capitated enrollees, without being at risk to ensure that the providers honor their noncontracted desires. To add these elements into the contract would be an act of micromanagement, and fewer providers would willingly accept capitation if every action were to be so closely monitored.

The providers, on the other hand, are also absolved from a charge of deceptive practice. The providers were not responsible for the promotion campaigns and advertisements that may have connoted a higher degree of choice than members actually had. All they had accepted was capitated or subcapitated risk to provide for the medical and diagnostic/therapeutic needs of a defined group of members with full flexibility in subcapitating with others. Ethics would dictate that lying to members is wrong, but the providers are not legally obligated to inform members that they signed up with an HMO that heavily capitates. In doing so, the provider would have to inform the member what capitation and subcapitation mean, and would have to absorb the angry outburst that would likely follow once the member learns where his or her premium dollar really goes (see Chapter Four).

The Wellness Shell Game

As with the element of choice, consumers are not told the truth about wellness. Consumers may be told that their employer has signed up with a health maintenance organization for their healthcare benefit, but they are not told the extent to which health maintenance is an oxymoron in most nonstaff-model HMOs. HMOs that capitate measure their members' health on a community-rated basis, and it is at the community level that they are evaluated by the National Council on Quality Assurance and by "report cards" of HMO quality. However, knowing that a community of members has a healthiness rating of 2.7 or 3.5 is important for the HMO to promote itself in selling more premium, but it is of poor utility to providers at risk to manage the health of individual people; to consumers who might want to choose providers (see above) on the basis of their performance in managing wellness rather than their office's color scheme; and to providers interested in subcapitation who'd like some idea of the healthiness of a population for which they'd accept risk. The problem isn't that wellness isn't an important criterion, but that it is currently an unmanageable commodity that is poorly defined and standardized.

In my opinion, it is insane for a provider to accept capitated risk without any means to identify, manage, and enhance the health of a given population. Since providers are not given wellness profiles of individual people, and perhaps only given the medical records of the few members of the population that have previously sought care in addition to whatever industry report cards they might have related to their *overall* wellness performance, providers are stuck. They're stuck with capitated risk, perhaps at high stop-loss levels, and no information about inherent health risks of individuals and which members need tighter or looser health management. They're stuck with voluminous, and frequently useless, reports that demonstrate the HMO's accountability in providing very basic data but do nothing to improve the level of useful knowledge that providers can employ. Very few providers have attempted to create a level of basic knowledge about inherent member health risks (by individual), short-term forecasting of resources needed to manage the risk they have, long-term strategizing to be less vulnerable when it is time for contract renegotiation, and what their ambulatory outcomes are for the members they are capitated/subcapitated to manage. When providers realize that there is a certain level of information unavailable to manage wellness (it is not told to providers by the HMO or by subcapitating providers), they move on to manage what they know they have: costs.

This is not to say that HMOs feel they've done their duty in managing the health of their subscribers. Staff-model HMOs have much more information about enrollees' health and provide far more opportunities for members to receive wellness-based care. Yet I know of very few such HMOs that utilize their wellness information about enrollees to tailor a wellness-enhancement program to which they can adhere. These HMOs have the common computer system and database management software to track and monitor enrollee health enhancement progress, should they desire to change. So far, however, these HMOs are being very selective in using this capability, even for chronically ill populations that could benefit from Disease State Management® education and training (see Chapter Five).

The message is loud and clear: HealthNet advertises in California with billboards of smiling people (typically children) that have the tag line "Well. Well. Well." Blue Cross of California's former HMO subsidiary (in a second incarnation) was called WellPoint. Many other examples of the misuse of "wellness" abound in every industry magazine and journal. The implication of all of those examples is that HMOs provide wellness to their members. But capitated members not part of staff-model HMOs typically don't receive wellness-oriented services tailored to their individualized health improvement.

Co-Provider Interrelationships

Members are also not told of the nature of the relationship between their chosen provider (see above) and their chosen hospital. In most cases, the HMO has so far paid capitation to both the selected gatekeeper group or IPA as well as to the chosen hospital or MCO. Members are not informed of the relationship between the two entities they've chosen to "patronize." Most members, if asked point-blank, would perceive that the gatekeeper is "on staff" with the HMO and/or is an exclusive provider to (some feel the provider is salaried by) the chosen hospital. Many members of HMOs are truly shocked to learn that the chosen providers typically fight with one another; in fact, there is general distrust between the parties and a pervasive seige mentality.

The facts of the matter are that hospitals need to ask the permission of the gatekeeper in order to treat his or her patient. There are often hard feelings between the two when the gatekeeper has limited office hours and unchecked voice mail or a malfunctioning answering machine during nights and weekends. At the same time, some providers persist in "gaming" the system by sending after-hour emergencies to the hospital emergency department for care, and sometimes second-guessing and/or denying emergency department personnel from payment for conditions which turn out to have been non-emergent all along. Hospitals are stuck because 24-hour emergency departments that accept Medicare (most every one) are required by law to treat and stabilize every patient who comes through their doors, and to assume every case is life-threatening until proved otherwise; the ill feelings surface because emergency departments can jeopardize the Medicare and Medicaid certification of the entire hospital including $50,000 fines if even one patient is turned away without initiating life-threat diagnostics (such as an HMO patient who was "turfed" to the emergency department without an obvious life-threatening condition, but the department pays a huge price for making an assumption that turns out to be wrong). The gatekeeper, particularly if the budget is tight, can "game" the hospital by retroactively denying emergency treatment based on the hindsight that the condition proved to be non-emergent. The result, for relative pennies of cost savings, is a feud between the gatekeeper and the hospital, even if both parties are capitated for the same patient!

Existence of Capitation

Members are kept in total darkness about capitation, subcapitation, and the implications of this form of health payment. Many providers in immature capitation markets do not truly understand the concept and the implications; in fact, many hospitals are unclear, perhaps due to jargon and ego (see Chapter Two) and perhaps due to the lack of measurable change that occurred following DRGs, a malady from which many MCOs still suffer. The emergence of capitation has blindsided many providers, virtually overnight. Few providers know what they would tell their patients (and enrollees) if questioned about standards and treatment implications related to capitation. To this issue, providers can breathe a sigh of relief: Members do not yet realize that there are issues, such as capitation and subcapitation, that fall through the cracks in their understanding of managed care.

The problem right now is that the knowledge of capitation, and how it has seriously compromised the ability of providers to manage the health and wellness of their contracted enrollees, is a bombshell. Without community-based transformation, as suggested by Dr. Tony Smith, knowledgeable consumers will have no means of moving forward in a capitated market, especially in so many markets around the country that have 25 percent or higher capitated managed care penetration, and not when proposals for more widespread capitated Medicare Risk plans are being debated on Capitol Hill as a means of keeping the Medicare program from insolvency. Capitated managed care, according to most forecasters, will represent close to 80 percent of the healthcare marketplace by the year 2000. Capitation is profitable for HMOs and is making for profitable providers, too. Even with full knowledge, the next steps have to involve managing capitation risk (Chapters Four and Five) and transforming the practice of capitation in the future to yield opportunities for providers (Chapter Six) and vendors (Chapter Seven).

Chapter Four

Understanding and Minimizing Current Capitation Risk

Having presented the basics about capitation, how it has evolved, and how it defines the current marketplace, we will now explore ways that capitated risk can be managed in today's mature and immature markets. In other chapters, we will explore opportunities to enhance the profitability of capitation from the standpoints of new strategies to minimize risk (Chapter Five), opportunities for providers to maximize benefits (Chapter Six), and opportunities for vendors (nonproviders) to derive benefit from an increasingly capitated marketplace (Chapter Seven).

This chapter will help you improve your understanding of (1) capitated risk management strategies, with particular attention to the concepts of "good" and "bad" risk; (2) the changes that need to occur among providers in managing capitated risk; (3) the role of capitation-covered enrollees; and (4) how we may repair the degradation of market-based contractual relationships among medical providers, institutional providers, and health plans themselves. The degrading of these relationships is one key factor that has led to rationing-based approaches and management strategies that are preemptive in nature. The bottom line in these approaches, however, involves paradigms, that is, what sense you make out of the world around you.

PARADIGMS DEFINED

Our ability to minimize current risks associated with capitation depends on our point of view. As with the question of whether the glass is half full or half empty, our perspectives of the marketplace can either enhance or constrain our approaches. With capitation, especially in mature markets where rationing-based approaches and the concept of "bad" risk are played out on a daily basis (see below), the perspective is very bleak and dismal. An example of this paradigm problem with capitation occurs among primary care groups receiving primary-only capitation (currently priced in Southern California within the $3 to $4 range): They perceive that they lose a lot of money on primary-only capitation, while recognizing that they must continue to contract for this business because they'd be bankrupt without it; to these physicians, capitation is a loser and any incremental cost—regardless of revenue offsets, incremental profit, or return on investment (ROI)—makes capitated business more of a loss. This paradigm plays out whenever a vendor comes to visit, offering new products to save money or software to better manage a population or costs associated with that population: Even if the total incremental cost is but one penny, the paradigm is that one more cent of cost is unacceptable for capitated business, regardless of any promised cost offset. This paradigm preserves a status quo that few feel requires preserving; because the perception is a paradigm, and no alternative paradigms have yet been presented (until now), groups of providers are mired in their faulty paradigms and have no option but to watch their businesses fail.

My view is that reality is static, but that the paradigms we use help define our perceptions of reality. For example, a provider whose paradigm suggested that capitation was a new form of reimbursement would continue his or her old behaviors of healthcare utilization based on a reimbursement mentality and would assume that pattern of utilization to be legitimate in a capitation era. Therefore, in this example, a consumptive attitude of healthcare under capitation (which could even remain static if such a provider were operating as part of an IPA that compensates on the basis of consumption and not on the basis of per member per month, or PMPM) is traced back to a faulty paradigm, not to the provider's misunderstanding or lack of familiarity with capitation. It is this very problem—well-taught providers operating in a vacuum that our own industry created and continues to support—that makes the study of paradigms so important for changing our perspectives of what is real and what is possible under capitated managed care. By the end of this book, I hope you'll share my view that our old paradigms related to capitation don't work because the basis for many of these paradigms was untrue from the outset.

We need to create new paradigms based on the reality of capitation, and to move away from the old paradigms we continue to believe. The first paradigm change that needs to occur is that providers and the public need to recognize that capitation is not a financial term but an operational term. The old paradigm is insidious because capitation came into being through the presentation by HMOs in the office of the chief financial officer. Capitation was a new form of payor contracting, the provider was told, whereby attractive funds could be offered prospectively to providers willing to assume more risk than under the status quo at that time. Now, in emerging and immature capitation markets, the same scenario is continuing to occur (which legitimizes a faulty paradigm creation): a new contract, new reimbursement, no contractual concessions, additional financial risk—all in the finance department of the provider, whether handled by the provider's accountant, controller, CFO, and/or director of contracting. The concept is presented as a financial change, requiring a financial response and strategy. The operational implications and tough changes in providers' operational behavior are never addressed, or suggested, because the original paradigm was a financial one.

Believing that capitation-related paradigms are financial in nature represents a no-win situation in any capitation market, emerging, immature, or mature. The financial mindset, of which I'm well aware, dictates that if revenues are going to become severely constrained, costs need to be cut back to the bone, all the more so if the revenue base is so low that current spending and operating levels cannot be maintained. The financial-based paradigm for a capitated enterprise attacks the causes of profit variance and is keyed to the assumption that capitation is wholly unprofitable and that cost management is the principal endeavor of the provider organization. This paradigm does not take into account what operating changes need to occur under capitation, but is fixated on what cost reductions need to occur to retain as much profit as possible. With no mind to influencing the directions of the business or to which enrollees seek care at what time and in what amount, the operation seeks to lose money on capitation and make the money back on volume.

And so the cycle begins: Add a capitation contract, assume more dilution of profit, and cut back to minimize profit dilution (with no end possible because there is no assumed profit in capitation from the outset); successful providers are deemed those whose enrollees don't generally complain, and the providers are invited to add additional contracts or have an edge in gaining additional contracts that they self-initiate. Unsuccessful providers are those whose enrollees become dissatisfied and either complain loudly or choose another provider while complaining loudly, resulting in their being dropped by health plans and/or their seeking cut-rate subcapitation from other providers (at even higher marginal cost and even lower profitability potential). In either cycle, new rounds of cost-cutting and the implications of such "knifings" are common elements within the financially oriented paradigm of capitation. In both cycles, there is no proactive attention paid to the enrollee except as a negative: damage control if the enrollee complains loudly to the HMO, especially so if the complaints are directed to the people at the health plan who contract with providers.

AN OPERATIONALLY DEFINED PARADIGM FOR CAPITATION

As a viable alternative to the no–win strategies and paradigms that accompany a financial-based approach, I would like to posit an operationally defined paradigm for capitation:

> Capitation is the means by which providers, either as contracting or subcontracting entities, assume outsourced responsibility from payors to manage the wellness of populations for whom a level of risk is borne; in so doing, capitated providers help individual members of such populations understand their roles and responsibilities under capitated managed care and provide supportive and nonpunitive guidance for such individuals to take responsibility for their own health status and that of their families.

This definition, until now unexpressed in even mature capitated markets, is a purely operational one. It focuses on the mechanisms by which capitated entities provide managed care, health maintenance, and wellness assurance to outsourced populations; it presumes that capitation has already occurred and recognizes that providers are looking to manage care and go into capitated arrangements to do so; and it provides guidance for providers interested in managing capitated populations (either by themselves or by others). In short, this definition represents a substantial paradigm shift in the emerging field of capitated managed care.

This paradigm shift is best appreciated when one considers what has previously passed for an understanding of capitated managed care. Other than this new definition, every classical definition of capitation expresses the relationship between provider and enrollee in financial terms: the nature of the per member per month (PMPM) relationship in setting dollar amounts, the inclusions/exclusions of populations subject to PMPM pricing, the variability of PMPM prices, the variability of risk assumption in setting PMPM prices, the method of indexing PMPM prices (if any), and the terms of contracted PMPM prices. The fallacy is that the definitions that dwell on the financial issues of capitation represent the *means* by which capitation occurs and do nothing to indicate *why* capitation is offered, *why* capitation is accepted, and *how* those who accept capitation make it successful for them. Thus, a financial paradigm in defining capitation never defines capitation in a meaningful way. A parallel can be drawn to describing a sport in terms of the financial arrangements between owners and players or how player agents get the best deals for their clients. Who could really understand a sport from its financial definition without having an objective description of the sport itself, especially a description of why participants would *want* to play the sport as well as how successful participants "win"?

Consumers tend to participate in managed care products, including capitated ones, due to a perception of lower cost reflecting moderate to good value. Payors participate in capitation because they are able to generate a substantial profit through outsourcing, in many cases at a higher level than they were able to generate through self-managed operations. Providers participate in capitation because they perceive that they must do so to survive, especially in developing and mature capitation markets; they participate in capitation only according to their specific risk assumptions.

A related phenomenon is that consumers are so poorly educated about appropriate healthcare consumption and healthcare providers that their expectations related to "value" are quite minimal. For example, consumers rate a hospital's quality not on the basis of its clinical outcomes, the board certification status of its physicians, its nosocomial infection rate (infections developed secondary to surgical procedures), or its morbidity and mortality statistics; instead, some customers tend to judge hospital quality based on cleanliness of public rooms and corridors, appropriate temperature of food, waiting time in the emergency department, and how many rings from a patient call button are needed to summon a nurse to a patient's room. When it comes to fixing value associated with capitated relationships, assumed value may be what an HMO tells the customer that value is rather than a customer's preconceived notions of value, especially for those new to HMOs in general. For existing customers of HMOs, value might be defined in the length of time a physician spends with a patient, the relative ease in scheduling appointments, and the promptness of returned phone calls; for the most part, consumers are not now fixing value of HMO coverage on the basis of industry report cards, the reliance of a network on IPAs instead of medical groups, or the use of clinical practice and wellness management parameters.

CURRENT PROVIDER RISK ASSUMPTIONS

There are currently three provider risk assumption strategies operating in capitated markets: the strategy of "good risk," the strategy of "bad risk," and the strategy of fence-sitters who have not yet decided which strategy to undertake or are unaware that they must, at some point, choose a single risk assumption strategy. (It should be noted that risk assumption strategies are also related to inherent flaws in the way capitation arrangements are made and priced, which are discussed in detail in Chapter Six.) The fence-sitters typically comprise new entrants to the managed care marketplace, such as a new IPA or other newly formed group that accepts subcapitation which is, at some point in an often complex contracting scheme, tied to a particular HMO. Thus, for example, a group of family practitioners might accept subcapitation for primary care services without formulating a specific contracting strategy for how they will define their business and marketing opportunities over the next three to five years; in the interim, they are merely participating in a capitated arrangement that, at some undecided later point, will result in more or fewer such arrangements. While these fence-sitters are part of the fabric of a capitated marketplace, they are in a temporary position. Market forces such as higher vendor costs, increases in covered lives who "drop plan" (either change employers or change insurance carriers/insurance products, which results in lower capitation fees), and/or reductions in negotiated PMPM prices offered by the seller will force the fence-sitters to take that "good hard look" which results in choosing either the good-risk or the bad-risk strategy. The good hard look will also convince some fence-sitters that they cannot compete on price and that they might have to choose between staying in business in an inhospitable market (such as joining increasingly intense competition for a shrinking pool of indemnity and FFS-paid business), being acquired by a large market force, going bankrupt, or supporting completely new capitation dynamics (see Chapter Six).

The best analogy for the good-risk and bad-risk strategies is investing in the commodities market, where the strategies are selling "short" (short-term profitability) and selling "long" (long-term profitability). The short market investment method (similar to my bad-risk strategy) is one where investors look for immediate paybacks on investments and intend on remaining in the market for a short time only. According to this strategy, if the market drops precipitously, the wise investor will try to get out with as many of his or her assets intact as possible. Let's consider this short-term strategy in further detail before evaluating the opposite strategy.

Bad Risk

According to the bad-risk strategy, providers look to capitation as a short-term positioning strategy to accomplish any or all of the following:

- *The "buy-me" strategy*—Control enough covered lives as quickly as possible, followed by forming an MSO as quickly as possible, to make the medical group attractive for purchase by a PHO, an acquiring medical group, or some other physician-acquisition venture.
- *The "commercial transformer" strategy*—Control enough capitation business directly from an HMO (in an immature capitation market) to become part of the first wave of distributors in an emerging subcapitation market.
- *The "conventional profiteering" strategy*—Differentiate on price and convenience in the subcapitation market (in a mature capitation market, and especially in critical specialties) to generate as much profit as possible in a not-yet-saturated subcapitation marketplace.
- *The "niche transformer" strategy*—Control enough niche, noncommercial capitation business directly from an HMO (in emerging second-wave markets where commercial capitation business is at or approaching saturation) to become part of the first wave of distributors in an emerging subcapitation market, examples including Medicare Risk, Medicaid, Workers Comp, and Disease State Management® markets.
- *The "niche profiteering" strategy*—Differentiate on price and convenience in niche subcapitation markets (in second-wave markets where commercial capitation business is already saturated), and especially in critical specialties, to generate as much profit as possible in a not-yet-saturated niche subcapitation marketplace.

The basic premise in these bad-risk strategies is that handling capitated business oneself for any length of time is unthinkable and generally undesirable. This premise also follows in the footsteps of the managed care plans themselves in that they were not organized to manage medical risk effectively. The HMOs' rush to outsource medical and institutional risk via capitation is reflective of a bad-risk strategy.

A corollary theory is that the provider can't reprice risk so low that no one buys it, because the provider doesn't want to get stuck holding on to that business. An example is the tertiary capitation business, where regional referral and academic medical centers offer PMPM "insurance" to other capitated providers to insulate against high-end risk like heart surgery; tertiary cap pricing is usually under $1 PMPM. The way the bad-risk games are played is similar to the children's game called "hot potato": Whoever is stuck holding on to capitated business when the music stops loses or is otherwise prevented from making a decent profit. The number of providers playing the bad-risk game determines how quickly capitated markets become saturated; how much price erosion occurs in both capitation- and subcapitation-based PMPM rates; how quickly second-wave markets emerge; and how long players remain in the market, either achieving their particular objectives or, like the short-market investor, getting out while remaining as financially unscathed as possible.

One of the realities of this corollary is that there is not enough price sensitivity experience yet in mature capitation markets to benchmark a parity level on capitation rates. For example, how can a provider know if a PMPM is "too high" if the bottom of the capitation market has not yet been reached? In Southern California in mid-1995, the bottom of the capitation market—either for primary or specialty capitation/subcapitation—has yet to level off.

In some cases, the bottoming-out in Southern California's subcapitation market is occurring by providers contracting for non-indexed capitation rates. What this means is that PMPM is not used as an indexing or adjustment mechanism for the rates themselves. The trend at the bottom of the market is to contract with a primary or specialty care IPA or provider group for a flat fee that is earmarked by the selling provider to "spend" on a capitated population. Thus, if $50,000 exists in the annual budget for servicing a population with no fluctuation possible, a purchaser of the subcapitated risk must agree to manage that risk for under the budgeted amount, in this case $50,000. The important piece here is that the $50,000 payment is a very fixed revenue not tied to any single health plan: The same $50,000 capitation is paid whether one hundred covered lives seek care or whether one million covered lives seek care. Without a strategy to manage that risk or to resell such bad risk, a subcapitating provider via fixed fee arrangements is taking a very expensive gamble.

Good Risk

The good-risk strategy is not unlike that of the long-market investor, who remains in the market to achieve long-range returns on investment. The long-market investor is fundamentally different from the short-market investor because he or she has enough assets to weather short-duration drops in the market for a particular commodity with the knowledge/hope that a long-range expectation will compensate for short-term fluctuations. The long-market investor is closely matched to providers practicing the good-risk strategy, who have long-range expectations that govern their participation in capitation and subcapitation markets notwithstanding infrequent "bad months" where performance is off-budget, earnings are diluted, or the combined operation is less than fully profitable (such as the first few months following an acquisition). Most MCOs are large enough to participate in the good-risk capitation contracting strategy.

According to the good-risk strategy, providers look to capitation as a long-term positioning strategy to accomplish either (and sometimes both) of the following:

- *The "HMO-buster" strategy*—Control enough covered lives (at least 100,000) within a broad enough geographic base that includes medical, nonmedical, and institutional providers—as quickly as possible—to enable the operation to apply to be a federally qualified HMO (FQHMO) and to apply for state licensure to sell premium to employers in return for customized health benefits; or make the medical group attractive for purchase by a PHO, an acquiring medical group, or some other physician acquisition venture.

- *The "No Lose" strategy*—Control enough covered lives (at least 100,000), differentiated on quality of health and services, within a broad enough geographic base that includes medical, nonmedical, and institutional providers—as quickly as possible—to improve contractibility with HMOs, and leave open the possibility of engaging in the HMO-buster strategy if HMO contracts fail to meet strategic and budgetary goals. This strategy is the one chosen by most MCOs.

The basic premise in these good-risk strategies is that capitation business is a desirable commodity. Given this premise, providers who believe in the good-risk strategy seek to differentiate themselves among other capitated providers on the basis of quality processes, attractive physical plant, good clinical outcomes, high customer satisfaction, and excellent customer service and convenience. These providers are investing in decision support and integrated computer systems and are seeking unique partnerships with vendors and other providers, especially those interested in bearing risk. These providers are developing the infrastructure and subsystems to manage risk effectively and are in the market for absorbing other capitated contracts, whether on a primary, subcap, or tertiary cap basis.

CURRENT CONTRACTUAL RELATIONSHIPS
BETWEEN PAYORS AND PROVIDERS

Because Southern California–style managed care defines itself according to its contractual relationships, particularly its capitated ones, suffice it to say that capitation-based contracting in a mature capitation market such as this one is quite volatile, especially at the time of this writing. As the capitation market becomes even more saturated, and as HMOs have stopped negotiating new commercial and Medicare Risk capitation agreements in such markets, the compression of the subcapitation marketplace among providers is particularly acute. With more cutthroat contracting practices, both in the good-risk and bad-risk scenarios, the marketplace is seeing increasingly creative means of packaging and reselling capitated risk among providers. Even tertiary capitation is starting to be resold. With no end in sight as of this writing, one of the commonalities in Southern California that can be observed, so far, is that sellers in these "subcapitation price wars" under the bad-risk strategy are generating lower profits than their subcapitators (meaning the ones who sold them the subcapitated risk they are now trying to resell) probably generated and are able to sell less-than-entire amounts of risk (meaning that buyers are choosing lower stop-loss rates to insulate themselves from unmanageable risk and/or that buyers want the seller to continue to assume certain administrative responsibilities). In turn, buyers in today's market are making lower-than-budgeted concessions on price in order to control ever-shrinking amounts of specialty medicine market share but at a lower risk profile (see above), which is partly reflective of lower subcapitation prices, and mostly reflective of the fact that *the gatekeeping model doesn't work,* especially for populations who are *known* to be unhealthy.

In Southern California, HMO premiums on the "open market" (exclusive of subsidizations by employers) are sufficient enough to generate very substantial profits for the HMO, but they squeeze providers, especially institutions, in return. (See table on page 85.) HMOs tend to cherry-pick populations on the basis of inherent health to the greatest possible extent. Even with premiums at the $600 level per month for family coverage (assuming a family is comprised of two adults and two children living in the same household), HMOs either will tend to deny coverage for preexisting conditions or, if prohibited from this practice by state regulations (which is becoming the case in California), will raise premiums far higher than this assumed level to include only wealthy individuals with one or more preexisting conditions.

Capitation 101 Income Statement
Just How Profitable and Where Does the Money Go?

Part I: The HMO

Revenue (annual premium payments per family = $7,200)

PMPM equivalent (Assuming $600/month and 4 members per family) ....$ 150

Expense (per family)

PMPM capitation to physicians (average 1993 Southern California rates; includes incentives, risk pools, administration, and education)   40

PMPM capitation to hospitals (average 1993 Southern California rates; includes incentive pool with physicians and risk pool)   40

Contribution Margin to HMO (for marketing, infrastructure, and profit) $ **70**

   % of Revenues (potential profit margin)   **47%**

Part II: The Full-Risk Physician Group/Panel

Revenue (from HMO, PMPM)...$ 40

Expense

Specialist risk pool allocation (@50% of revenue received)   20

   Less specialty subcapitations (assumed 50% of risk pool, expressed as aggregated PMPM)   10

   Net risk pool for noncapitated specialists (expressed as aggregated PMPM)   10

Primary care subcapitation (average 1993 Southern California PMPM)   5

Operating expenses (PMPM equivalent)   10

Contribution Margin to Physicians (potential profit, less incentives and noncapitated specialist exps) $ **15**

   % of Revenues (potential profit margin)   **38%**

Part III: The Full-Risk Hospital Provider

Revenue (from HMO, PMPM)...$ 40

Expense

Risk pool for other institutions (@50%; reflects that few institutional subcapitation arrangements were in place in Southern California in 1993)   20

Operating expenses (@ PMPM equivalent; e.g., obtaining authorizations, defending against retroactive denials)   15

Contribution Margin to Hospital (potential profit, less outliers & denied treatments) $ **5**

   % of Revenues (potential profit margin)   **13%**

Recap	
HMO profit potential per family per year	$3,360
Physicians' profit potential per family per year	720
Hospital's profit potential per family per year	240

In the wake of discounting that is occurring in sales to employers and large public employee consortia (such as the California Public Employees Retirement System, CAL-PERS), HMOs are embarking on their own form of cost shifting. Not unlike the practices that MCOs have utilized in the past, HMOs are employing cost-shifting techniques on two fronts to offset losses they incur from the "need" to discount premium heavily to large group employers and to wrestle market share among small group employers. First, premiums for the self-employed (who aren't a small group or don't qualify for small group coverage), for workers who decline limited health benefits offered by their employers (such as HMO coverage with limited provider panels that are inconvenient to where they live or work), for workers in very small businesses not required to offer health insurance to their employees, and for the unemployed are higher than premiums paid by employers and are escalated higher for preexisting conditions or for previous utilization of healthcare resources (such as seeing a physician or going to the hospital any time in the last seven years—this is not a joke—or for taking any prescribed drug). On the second front, definitions of preexisting conditions are unusually harsh for the self-employed, the working "refuseniks," disadvantaged workers, and the unemployed.

The term *preexisting conditions* under cost shifting has come to mean any rationale that the HMO can use to deny coverage to all but the healthiest or wealthiest individuals. HMOs typically deny coverage to individuals on the basis of being, or having been, a smoker; consuming any quantity of alcohol in a given week (this prohibition includes the "Saturday night beer" or even a single glass of wine); being more than 20 percent above one's ideal weight, even if one is only a couple of pounds above the threshold; or having a high cholesterol reading, as measured on either the total cholesterol, HDL cholesterol, LDL cholesterol, or triglycerides level. While these are generally acceptable, appropriate measures of good health, they are quite intrusive into what society generally considers to be liberties and are quite unrealistic to expect of people short of sainthood. For example, more than 50 percent of the U.S. population is more than 20 percent above their ideal weight, the clinical definition of obesity. In fact, one should consider the low likelihood of acceptance to HMO plans by these criteria when applicants who have truthfully disclosed that they have not been to a physician or a hospital in the last seven years (and, if so, will leave their entire medical history and medical record open to scrutiny for causes of denial—such as having an acute medical condition that required seeking medical care in the first place) will have had no benefit in improving their lifestyle based on previous testing and measurement of these conditions, at least within the last seven years. The real cost shifting is that those applicants who are accepted via this route will be the least risk-averse of any population insured by the HMO and the least likely to require consumption of provider services—in other words, the most profitable. This discrimination against the middle and lower middle classes explains why so many Americans lack health insurance.

HMO CONTRACTUAL RELATIONSHIPS UNDER CAPITATION

Referring to the Capitation 101 Income Statement on page 85, premium received from a family of four could be divided by 4 to approximate the PMPM equivalent of capitation-based premium. In this example, where $600 per family household is received per month as premium, the PMPM equivalent revenue would be $150. The $150 represents the total amount of revenues per member per month that the HMO can use to pay its capitation-related expenses, to pay its own overhead for the maintenance of capitation business (such as reinsurance coverage), and to contribute to its own profit.

Like any business, the HMO has expenses under capitation. The nature of the capitation relationship is that the HMO can offer a PMPM capitation payment to, if possible, a single medical group or, less preferably, a multispecialty IPA for full-risk medical coverage at as high a stop-loss level as the provider will accept. Some capitators (this term covers both HMOs selling capitation as well as providers offering subcapitation to other providers) will gauge a provider's willingness to accept high stop loss by providing differential capitation rates according to differential stop-loss levels accepted. For example, a capitator might offer $30 PMPM for $50,000 stop loss; $31.50 PMPM for $100,000 stop loss; and $33 PMPM for $250,000 stop loss. The willingness of the provider to accept modest increases in capitation for substantially higher stop loss tells a capitator much about the provider's operation and receptiveness to bearing risk, assuming of course that the provider understands the insurance business and his or her operation's capacity to bear risk in an appropriate and profitable manner.

An early 1990s price commonly paid in Southern California for full-risk medical capitation was about $40 PMPM. Full-risk medical capitation means any and all professional services consumed by a given population of capitated enrollees, whether such services are consumed by physicians who are members of the capitated group/IPA or who practice outside it. Such services include patient care done in a physician's office, in an urgent care center and/or clinic, in an institution (other than hospital charges exclusive of professional fees), or in any and all other medical or nonmedical settings, such as a chiropractor's office if chiropractic services are part of the HMO's stated coverage. Physicians receiving full-risk medical capitation therefore have an incentive to create as many sub-capitated relationships as possible to avoid having to pay many specialists on a DFFS basis, thus putting capitated physicians at risk for full-retail or slightly below-retail charges.

Institutional capitation is another expense historically borne by HMOs in sending enrollee populations to capitation. Although the early 1990s price commonly paid in Southern California for full-risk institutional capitation was about $40 PMPM, current trends are forcing full-risk medical and institutional providers to get by on far less combined capitation (see below). Full-risk institutional capitation involves providing for all nonmedical care rendered within the MCO's institutions *or in other institutions not part of the MCO*. For example, the care for a capitated enrollee who requires inpatient psychiatric care would be the responsibility of the MCO provider receiving institutional capitation for nonmedical services, whether or not such an institution is part of the MCO; in this example, if care is rendered within a psychiatric hospital not part of the managed care organization, the bill for any and all institutional services is sent to the MCO. Tertiary cap also falls into this category. Thus, the MCO retains more capitation dollar based on its breadth and depth of affiliations, and on its ability to enter into case rates—or, ideally, subcapitation—with external institutional providers on which the MCO must depend.

The financial impetus for HMOs to enter into full capitation arrangements, both medical and institutional, is to reduce their administrative expenses and effect savings in their own. In the days when HMOs were paying on FFS or DFFS, their infrastructure and infrastructure-related expenses were tremendous. Since the HMO was reimbursing providers on the basis of billed claims, the organizations required tremendous infrastructures to handle thousands of claims every day (e.g., storage, mail rooms, delivery personnel, trash management, computers, claims personnel, claims adjudication personnel, utilization review nurses or subcontracts for such services, and postage costs) to do a type of job they had little experience doing themselves. Where an HMO contracted with each pairing of professional service organization (for full-risk medical) with health service organization (for full-risk institutional), the HMO cut its infrastructure down from tens of thousands of claims paid to all providers each month to 24 checks a year: 12 checks to the capitated professional service organization and 12 checks to the capitated health service organization! This change in contracting has freed HMOs to do what they do best: sell premium.

The newest contracting trend, where allowed in very mature capitation markets, is to cut the infrastructure back from 24 checks per year (to two providers) to 12 checks per year (to a single "superprovider"). This trend, unimaginatively called *full-risk capitation* is different from full-risk medical capitation and from full-risk institutional capitation. The term *full-risk capitation* (albeit sometimes confused with the lesser forms of capitation) is given to very large medical providers with sufficient depth and breadth of coverage (controlling at least 100,000 covered lives) at an amount equal to the full-risk medical capitation plus somewhere between 50 and 75 percent of the standard full-risk institutional capitation rate, based on an assumption of a benefit from economies of scale and the reduced need to duplicate each other's services in order to manage capitated business.

In the Capitation 101 example, full-risk capitation might have been offered (had it existed) in the early 1990s at about the $60 to $70 PMPM level. The current pricing trend is in response to heavy premium discounting during the last three open enrollment periods, especially so in Southern California. Since the HMOs are experiencing limited price elasticity (meaning that they are unable to do conventional cost shifting by increasing premium prices), their strategy has been to cut PMPM rates by about 15 to 20 percent overall (meaning that a mid-1990s adjustment to full-risk capitation rates to supergroups might be as low as $48 to $56 PMPM). The effect on the HMO would be to increase PMPM profit to $100 (a 67 percent margin)!

Unfortunately, the bottom has not yet dropped out of the Southern California market. Full-risk medical capitation prices in early 1995 are under $30 PMPM; on the specialty side, there are dermatology panels accepting subcapitation rates in Southern California as low as 23 cents PMPM and neurology groups accepting subcap at 18 cents PMPM. Primary care commercial capitation rates are well below $4 PMPM, meaning that providers engaging in the bad-risk scenario who have received primary-only subcapitation at $5 to $6 are enjoying a fantastic windfall, all assuming that such subcapitating primary care physicians (PCPs) provide quality care (or have subcapitated to a group that does) and remain financially solvent. While these rates may seem low, many PCPs can manage risk effectively at these prices; yet these providers have no margin for error of any kind, which is exacerbated if the level of information from the subcapitating provider (if any) is less than complete and accurate.

The $70 contribution margin to the HMO is not viewed by health plans as complete profit, because it doesn't include marketing expenses and administrative infrastructure expenses. In addition, since HMOs have multiple product offerings of which capitation is a part, any capitation product profits will be used by such health plans to offset other product losses, such as PPO and indemnity coverage. Since HMOs are not required to disclose their financial performance by product, it has been rare to find a double- or triple-option HMO with a reported combined profit margin much above 10 percent.

On the other hand, the majority of the $70 should be viewed as true profit to the HMO, even if the HMO accounts for it differently. The reason for viewing such contributions to income as profit is that they are monies derived from outsourcing. With medical and institutional care outsourced, including allowances for reinsurance liability—reflecting either high capitation rates if all or substantially all reinsurance liability is assumed or low rates if substantial reinsurance liability is not assumed, which allows for paying for that coverage plus a profit margin—and perhaps some administrative expenses (such as claims management, claims adjudication, and coordination of member benefits), any remaining expenses do not reflect expenses that need to be incurred by the HMO *for that family.* The infrastructure and marketing expenses noted in the Capitation 101 table under HMO Contribution Margin are incurred to sell new premium, to create new outsourced relationships, and to generate incremental HMO profit.

For example, a billboard promoting the HMO or HMO product seen by motorists in a given market area might generate increased membership in an area that is already capitated—resulting in an adjustment to the number of members for which capitated providers receive funds but *not* changing the PMPM rates—and might generate increased membership in unsubscribed or uncapitated areas. The latter scenario is more likely because the HMO does market research in deciding on where billboards are to be placed (ostensibly to generate greater return on investment per advertising dollar paid) and on the sales message contained on each billboard. The promotion return on investment that an HMO would use to justify spending money on a billboard involves either signing up a new employer group (incremental capitation), enticing large numbers of employees to choose that HMO over other HMOs during an open enrollment period (incremental capitation), and/or enticing large numbers of employees to choose that HMO over other health insurance options during an open enrollment period (also incremental capitation). In short, HMOs promote themselves to generate premium, which—according to the Capitation 101 Income Statement—provides the working capital to fund new capitation arrangements. The numbers of commercial capitation subscribers, which are increased through the successful investment in advertising, become a basis for selling additional Medicare Risk subscriptions, which leads to additional capitation arrangements substantially more profitable than commercial capitation.

MEDICAL PROVIDERS' CONTRACTUAL RELATIONSHIPS UNDER CAPITATION

Referring to the Capitation 101 Income Statement on page 85, full-risk *medical* capitation received from the managed care plan (in this example, $40 PMPM) provides the revenue basis for the medical group or IPA. It is on the basis of this PMPM amount that medical providers budget for their capitated business. Even though these providers collect on minimal co-payments at the time of service ($2 to $20 per ambulatory care visit), this revenue is applied as a contra-expense—in other words, an offset against consumption-related expenses incurred per ambulatory care visit. Additionally, because co-payment revenues are dependent on consumption—the antithesis of successful capitation—medical providers budget based solely on their contracted PMPM revenues. The PMPM itself, in this case $40, becomes the sole revenue against which fixed and variable expenses are paid.

On the expense side, a medical provider has at least four types of expenses, which are incurred either internally or externally: risk pool–related expenses; subcapitation expenses (typically 90 to 100 percent of primary care and 50 percent or more of specialty care, as much as possible); insurance expenses; and internal infrastructure-related expenses. The types of external expenses might include other medical providers, MCOs and other healthcare institutions, home healthcare providers, and other vendors and institutions.

Under FQHMO guidelines for commercial capitation, a capitated provider under full-risk medical must set aside 50 percent of capitation revenues as a risk pool, a reserve against out-of-network specialty care that covered lives may require. Using the Capitation 101 Income Statement as a guide, and assuming that the terms are applied to a population of 10,000 covered lives, the medical group would set aside $200,000 each month into the risk pool ($40 × 10,000 × 50%). The risk pool's value at the end of the year would be $2.4 million (200,000 × 12), plus carryover, if any, from prior year(s), less specialty claims presented to the medical providers for payment during that period. The concept behind the risk pool concept is that well-managed medical providers responsible for the medical risk of *generally healthy enrollees* will consume less than 50 percent of capitation revenues for specialty care.

The FQHMO guidelines, however, do not specify what constitutes sound medical provider management under capitation nor what benchmarking the federal government did to arrive at the 50 percent ratio; instead, the guidelines were strictly financial standards tied to assumptions of adequate cash flow and not to an appropriate management of operational infrastructure or actual medical practice. The result is that under-capitalized groups remain untrained in proper operations management, let alone necessary wellness management techniques (including Disease State Management®) for capitated populations. What passes for management for these medical providers is risk pool preservation by ensuring that no more than 50 percent of monthly capitation revenue is spent for specialty care. Without necessary management tools to allocate resources intelligently and to reduce demands for consumption, these providers merely deny as many demanded consumption requests as possible, hoping that as much of the risk pool can be retained as income each month— in other words, they ration care for healthy people.

Medical providers involved in capitated relationships usually try to avoid the stigma associated with rationing. Like the large amount of would-be restaurateurs who end up selling or foreclosing within their first year of operations, many medical providers who go into capitation espousing one of the good-risk strategies end up changing to a bad-risk strategy after being burned for the first few months due to undercapitalized risk pools. Their patients come to conclude that their physicians are insensitive to appropriate diagnosis and to appropriate treatment of their medical conditions when the medical providers blatantly ration. Ration-based operations represent one of the chief sources of complaints to HMOs, regulators, and anyone else who will listen. Oddly, most medical providers see themselves as being forced to ration, believing that they have no other operational strategies and knowing that they lack the infrastructure to do anything differently if they were educated as to the tricks of the trade (see Chapter Five).

One of the strategies medical providers employ to reduce their need to ration, regardless of their risk strategy, is to enter into subcapitation arrangements with specialists. Using the 10,000 covered lives example against a $40 monthly rate for full-risk medical capitation, obstetrical care could be subcapitated for $1.85 PMPM. The impact of this subcapitated rate is that members of a full-risk medical group could insulate themselves from routine obstetrical care that 10,000 individuals might demand for $18,500 per month (within contracted corridors of liability that are reflective of the reinsurance contract that the seller negotiated with the HMO). By comparison, a single vaginal delivery by an obstetrician might cost $1,000 on a DFFS basis; a single C-section delivery by an obstetrician might cost $3,000 via DFFS. Therefore, subcapitation is an important component of the field of capitation. For medical providers practicing the good-risk strategy, subcapitation contracting is motivated more by those who can help provide a value-added benefit to full-risk providers, enhancing the way they practice and the way they deliver high quality per capitation dollar received. By contrast, medical providers practicing the bad-risk strategy enter into subcapitation contracts motivated more by price; in other words, subcapitation allows them to allow subcontractors to accept blocks of risk at prices lower that what they can accept themselves or what they can sell to anyone else.

The HCFA requirement that 50 percent of HMO-paid capitation must be accrued to a risk pool is a highly variable expense, especially if out-of-network providers submit bills to the capitated physicians for services rendered, whether paid via FFS, DFFS, or some form of "per case" contract. Given this reality, subcapitation could be used to reduce the exposure such physicians could have from consumption-based contracting by making the risk pool less variable and therefore more "fixed." As a general rule, then, subcapitation is a strategy that medical providers utilize to make their risk pools less variable. The more subcapitation they can negotiate with specialists (whether or not it is appropriate to do so), the less consumption-based exposure they face. The goal for bad-risk players is to approach 100 percent subcapitation to specialists for risk pooling; the goal for good-risk players is to have as much specialty care as possible done within the group or within a defined network, with whatever out-of-network specialty care done on as close as possible to a 100 percent sub-capitated basis (negotiated on a combination of price, patient care performance, and clinical outcomes—a *value* basis). An aggregated average of subcapitation, reflecting both good-risk and bad-risk provider strategies, is approximately 50 percent of total risk pool allocation.

Perhaps the centerpiece of medical provider capitation relationships is gatekeeping. The need for gatekeeping, especially in commercial capitation, presumes that, generally, *populations are healthy* and do not need to see a physician. Hence, gatekeeping is needed to restrict care to healthy people. Because capitated managed care involves the creation of gatekeepers to manage populations, responsibility typically rests with primary care physicians, also known as PCPs. Medical providers who are more than 50 percent dependent on capitated revenues are tending to shy away from general practitioners (GPs) as gatekeepers due to increasing questions about medical safety, medical risk, and quality. While there are many high-quality GPs practicing in gatekeeper arrangements, both payors and quality-minded medical provider groups are now favoring board-certified "specialties" such as family practice, pediatrics, internal medicine, and obstetrics/gynecology, with liberal use of physician extenders such as registered nurse practitioners and physician assistants. In the most mature capitation markets, we are observing some compression in the use of internists and OB/GYNs as PCPs, especially as more medical school graduates are choosing family medicine over the surgical specialties and subspecialties and as more positions previously held by physicians are being filled by extenders who can diagnose [such as Registered Nurse Practitioners (RNPs) and Physician Assistants (PAs)]. Additional compression is occurring in these markets among OB/GYNs, especially because family practitioners and their extenders can deliver low- to medium-risk babies and because infertility care, the chief revenue generator among FFS OB/GYN practices, is frequently not a covered benefit of HMO policies. In addition, perinatologists are sent referrals of high-risk mothers and pediatricians are called in when there are indications at the time of labor that the baby is distressed or if a high-risk mother delivers via Caesarean. Thus, physician practitioners within mature capitation markets have redefined referral and practice patterns that are serving to obviate the needs for certain medical specialties such as obstetrics.

PRIMARY CARE AND GATEKEEPING EXPENSES

The term *gatekeeping* is in my opinion derogatory, especially in how it is being applied in capitated markets. The term implies that members seeking care are so unknowledgeable about appropriate and inappropriate usage of managed care resources that they *need* to be monitored and supervised by the physician. This rationale might apply to healthy people, but the vast majority of the U.S. population is far from healthy, requiring a new capitation system (see Chapter Six). If personalized monitoring and supervising were, in fact, occurring, capitated markets would be much different than they are today. The reason for this difference is that gatekeeping is assumed to be synonymous with financial accountability, cost-cutting, and rationing. The troublesome undercurrent is that there is no trust built into the system—that true gatekeeping can, at some point, become obsolete when consumers and physicians are properly trained to consume managed care resources appropriately and when consumers, with the guidance of their physicians and extenders, are allowed to take responsibility for their own lifestyles and for their own resultant health status. Gatekeeping is viewed today as a necessary, permanent centerpiece of capitation, like the central cog of the great gearbox of managed care, instead of a temporary measure until the marketplace, as a whole, matures in its views and attitudes toward capitated managed care.

Referring back to the Capitation 101 Income Statement, the role of gatekeeping is a universal cost among capitated medical providers. Among medical providers practicing the good-risk strategy, primary care is a commodity that is often retained by the group or IPA because it is so central to the group's success or failure and to both ambulatory clinical outcomes as well as overall consumer satisfaction. Even the smallest groups practicing the good-risk strategy invest in the infrastructure to self-manage primary care, including urgent care, diagnostic ancillar services (e.g., laboratory, radiology, and noninvasive cardiovascular services), minor surgery (including colorectal diagnostics and suturing/splinting), and high-exposure therapeutic services (such as physical therapy and pharmacy). Thus, for good-risk providers, primary care gatekeeping becomes an expense borne by their own infrastructure and is typically not subcapitated to others.

Subcapitation of primary care is a centerpiece of medical providers practicing the bad-risk strategy. If a medical provider's risk strategy is to become insulated from capitated risk, primary care gatekeeping becomes the first service to go. Some of the quickest market price compression occurs in subcapitating for primary care services. A market price for primary care subcapitation in Southern California in the early 1990s was $6 to $7.50 PMPM; as of this writing in mid-1995, the average price (if available) is between $3 and $4 PMPM. In 1993, the aggregated average PMPM for primary care subcapitation was about $5.

On these kinds of margins, PCPs are hard-pressed to provide any value-added services for their covered lives. These PCPs frequently scramble to satisfy the seemingly endless stream of covered lives who present themselves for treatment in their offices, because—since they advocate a bad-risk strategy—they lack the infrastructure investments to manage their populations and manage them in ways that are not dependent on seeing patients in their office or clinic. In addition, many of the "bottom-feeding" PCPs buying subcapitated risk that may have been resold at least two or three times may themselves be fence-sitters (see p. 80), which poses additional coverage risks for a subcapitating medical provider group or IPA, especially if the PCPs decide not to stay in business or in a practice that decides to remain heavily involved in capitated managed care for an extended period of time.

OTHER FULL-MEDICAL RISK EXPENSES

Among capitated medical providers, the portion of capitation received representing the net of risk pool allocations and subcapitation paid, if any, is used to cover their own operating expenses as well as to cover any claims that may be required by out-of-network providers against a risk pool that was depleted during that month. Any amount of money remaining after covering operating expenses and risk pool shortfalls becomes the pre-tax net income of the medical provider group. The amount of the contribution margin paid to physician partners or owners of the medical group represents a potential profit; the actual profit retained by the group is the difference between this potential profit and any physician incentives that may need to be paid to group members practicing good managed care medicine or attaining group-budgeted targets for certain high-cost, consumer-satisfaction-reducing, or quality- or safety-compromising procedures. The average contribution margin among physicians receiving full-risk medical capitation from HMOs was about 38 percent in the early 1990s.

From an operating expense standpoint, the infrastructure expenses are the last to be paid because subcapitation expenses, if any, are the first to be paid. This reality is the case regardless of a good-risk or bad-risk capitation strategy: Subcapitation, depending on how value is measured (e.g., price alone or incremental quality, service, and price in combination), is a desirable delegation of responsibility that can be compromised if subcapitated fees are not paid. Thus, subcapitation becomes an insurance policy that no provider wants to let lapse.

The $15 contribution margin to the medical provider is much further from "true" profit as can be assumed for the HMO. The contribution margin that physicians in capitated and subcapitated arrangements receive is less completely linked to profit because of the need to pay noncapitated specialist fees, which can very easily surpass risk pool reserves, especially in the first 18 months of accruals. In addition, incentive compensation is typically earmarked against contribution margins.

The kicker about medical providers' contribution margins is that much (if not all) of the incentive compensation is *promised* to the members of a medical group as a bonus for practicing good managed care medicine; in reality, it is the medical group or IPA administrator(s) whose own incentive compensation is typically tied to the physician. The premise is that a group's owner's equity is shared by its owners but that retained risk pool earnings (in other words, the annual effect of less risk pool money going out than coming in) is as much a function of the contracting savvy of management than the physicians themselves. There is some truth to this premise, especially when one considers that the extent to which risk pool dollars are earmarked against subcapitation deals (that a group's vice president of contracting might negotiate on behalf of the organization), which reduce the variability of those funds. The subcapitating of risk pools gradually makes risk pool retained earnings more fixed, thus guaranteeing the group positive cash flow at year-end due not to the practice of good managed care medicine (as physicians have historically believed) but to savvy contracting practices that increasingly insulate medical groups and IPAs from variable risk.

INSTITUTIONAL PROVIDERS' CONTRACTUAL RELATIONSHIPS UNDER CAPITATION

Institutional providers, in emerging capitation markets, receive capitation directly from payors. This capitation comprises outsourced wellness management for enrollees utilizing health service organizations. The capitation covers such care as hospital room and board (known in the industry as daily hospital service or DHS); all diagnostic ancillary services (e.g., clinical and pathology laboratory, cardiovascular and cardiac catheterization laboratory, vascular laboratory, diagnostic imaging); all therapeutic ancillary services (e.g., pharmacy, intravenous therapy, physical and occupational therapy, respiratory therapy, acute dialysis, surgery); and institutional-related services that may be required outside the hospital (e.g., outpatient radiation therapy and chemotherapy, home health or hospice therapy, and home infusion therapy [such as respiratory and dialysis]). Institutional capitation also covers institutional care that might not be provided within a particular network but requires care from competitors, such as long-term care, tertiary or quaternary inpatient care (e.g., burn treatment and transplantation services). Tertiary Cap is offered for both tertiary care (e.g., open-heart surgery) and quaternary care (e.g., bone marrow transplantation).

In such emerging capitation markets, the flow of capitation from payor to institutional provider is depicted in the Capitation 101 Income Statement. The hospital provider receives PMPM revenue from the HMO and, like the medical provider, must earmark at least 50 percent to its own risk pool. This risk pool accrues funds to compensate other institutions (outside the institutional provider's defined network of institutions) for nonmedical care required for their covered population. For example, if a portion of a hospital's capitated population requires nursing home care following short institutional stays for cerebrovascular accidents (strokes), and the hospital lacks an appropriate supply of skilled nursing beds, it may be forced to send the patient to a freestanding nursing home in the community and compensate the provider out of its institutional risk pool. Except for a surprisingly few number of institutions that contract with quaternary medical centers for tertiary capitation (earmarking typically less than $1 PMPM for insulation against high-end risk), very little of institutional risk pool funds were spent in subcapitation arrangements in the early 1990s.

This low level of subcapitation by capitated institutional providers, especially as existed in Southern California in the early 1990s, is a marked contrast to the extent of subcapitating that was occurring among capitated medical providers during the same period. By the same token, most hospitals had deeper pockets than medical groups, and did not perceive that they were at as much risk for rapid risk pool depletion. Even today, very little—perhaps as much as 25 percent—of hospital risk pools is earmarked against subcapitated institutional relationships; this low level of subcapitation makes much more of the patient care costs associated with capitated revenues variable rather than fixed. The net effect, coupled with higher infrastructure expenses for managing capitated institutional business (e.g., obtaining authorizations from gatekeepers, collecting co-payments, coordinating enrollee benefits, providing for reinsurance coverage, and defending against retroactive denials made by capitated medical provider adjudicators or their agents) relative to the infrastructure expenses for managing capitated medical operations, is a much lower contribution margin of only 12½ percent, which reflects only $5 net income per $40 of capitated gross revenues.

The $5 contribution margin to the institutional provider is much further from "true" profit than that which can be assumed for the HMO, and even for the medical provider. The contribution margin that hospitals in capitated and increasingly subcapitated arrangements receive is less completely linked to profit because of the need to pay noncapitated institutional fees, with a single bone marrow transplant (BMT) of $250,000 easily wiping out an entire year's risk pool; it is unclear why, in Southern California for example, institutional providers would choose not to earmark 25 cents or so PMPM to insulate themselves from BMT liability by subcapitating with an academic medical center that sells tertiary capitation. In fact, because such risk is quaternary, geographic proximity need not be a factor in negotiating for such tertiary capitation.

A hidden cost to institutional providers receiving capitation is that most risk pool earnings are shared between the hospital and the medical provider responsible for gatekeeping for the shared population. In most cases, however, the rapid depletion of hospital risk pools due to inadequate levels of subcapitation results in very little net earnings, which must be shared with the medical provider. As hospitals are successful in subcapitating more of their institutional risk to others, and subcontracting institutions become more receptive and adept at accepting subcapitated institutional risk from MCOs, hospital risk pool earnings will increase and will yield incremental earnings to medical providers' capitated earnings. It is as yet unclear how much of such incremental earnings—when they are generated—will result in additional distribution to physician owners of capitated entities or will result in additional incentive compensation to the managers of such operations.

The bottom line of the Capitation 101 Income Statement is that HMOs receive their margins off the top in capitated relationships and that the 47+ percent contribution margin is closer matched to true profitability, given the outsourced product, than is true for the medical and institutional providers' corresponding contribution margins related to capitation. Another important point is that the net effect per family per year gives providers much less room for error, with medical providers having triple the leeway as institutional providers. For example, a hospital's profit potential per family per year of just $240 is so low that a single service adjudicated to be denied for payment can instantly eliminate any profit potential for that family. While a medical provider's profit potential per family per year is triple the institution's potential, the $720 margin doesn't go very far either, especially if there is any volume of specialist bills that remain on a noncapitated basis and are charged on DFFS. The real bottom line here is that the profit margins are much tighter for those who provide the care than for those who outsource it; this reality indicates an inherently flawed relationship because healthy people don't need medical and institutional specialty care (see Chapter Six). It should also be noted that providers' contribution margins increase to the extent that they subcapitate to others; in other words, providers become more profitable when they imitate outsourcing HMOs.

REEXAMINATION OF CONTRACTUAL RELATIONSHIPS UNDER CAPITATION

Contractual relationships under healthcare capitation have generally been limited to three players: payors representing managed care insurance plans, medical providers, and institutional providers. Emerging players starting in early 1994 began to include certain medical supply vendors and home health agencies, contracting with providers on a capitated basis; this trend, which I call *vendor capitation,* is slowly becoming more widespread and is discussed more completely in Chapter Seven. The remainder of this section concerns risk minimization strategies that traditional capitation players currently utilize.

Managed care plans recognize quite clearly how much money is to be made at capitation, especially while premiums have reached parity in many markets. Consider that the basis for the scope of HMO work (namely capitating healthcare instead of providing healthcare directly) has changed dramatically while the price of premiums has decreased nominally, but in effect remained roughly unchanged. In fact, premium prices paid by employers—HMOs' primary customers—have risen rather than fallen, and premium prices in given markets are roughly the same as those of other payors, including staff-model HMOs, which truly provide services themselves rather than capitate to others. What all of this means is that HMOs experience a windfall because premiums for capitated plans are dramatically over-priced given the scope of work involved—and customers keep buying.

It should be no surprise, therefore, that managed care plans in uncapitated or immature capitated markets are jealously eyeing the profitability of California HMOs and are looking to cash in as well. The problem, of course, is that their marketplaces are not yet ready to commence widespread capitation. I would argue, in fact, that the *marketplaces themselves* (providers, employers, employees, and customers) are not yet ready for capitation, regardless of how much profit potential capitation represents to these businesses.

What I see happening is that these managed care plans are trying to jump-start a rapid progression to capitation by providing seed money for physicians to form IPAs and medical groups, providing exclusive provider "franchises" for defined populations, and getting customers and providers to feel comfortable about participating in panel and group settings. The HMOs pay the providers on DFFS against overly generous UCRs; give the providers a *taste* of risk bearing by introducing the concept of case rates, perhaps tied to DRG case-mix indexes; and start enticing consumer loyalty with reduced paperwork, incorporating high-quality physicians and hospitals in developing networks and panels, and reduced out-of-pocket fees. The purpose of these initial inroads is not to generate a profit (that will definitely come later) but to build consumer loyalty and provider confidence. In the second phase, EPOs will be launched to tie in employer loyalty and PSPs will be marketed to lock in the most loyal managed care physicians, all the while using capitated fees and generous risk pools as incentives to the most loyal players. Once the loyalty is solidified, as has already happened in Southern California, the HMOs lower the boom and capitate entire markets to their most loyal (and most profitable) providers. Once commercial capitation is locked in, the HMOs proceed to generate enough covered lives, at the same time readying their applications to HCFA to begin offering Medicare Risk (where the *real* money is made).

The managed care plans are starting to realize that outsourcing healthcare has a real drawback: education. Education is the methodology by which wellness management, instead of illness treatment, occurs. The power of wellness education is diminished when providers are not given the tools to manage health and wellness appropriately, are not provided the right infrastructure to effect quality education at all, and are not made aware of their responsibilities to provide wellness education in the first place. While outsourcing risk is profitable, jeopardizing appropriate consumer education threatens the market security and market longevity of managed care plans, especially if new competitors can undercut HMO premium and be satisfied with 30 percent profit margins instead of 50 percent ones. A new era occurs when competitors to health plans can generate 100,000 covered lives and qualify with the appropriate state agencies to offer premium to employers. In this era, which includes not just FQHMOs but also providers licensed at the state level to compete with HMOs for selling premium, managed care plans must differentiate to retain market share. Educating members, on behalf of capitated providers, to change unhealthy lifestyles and to take responsibility for their health status represents a powerful differentiation factor in the upcoming years that will also help minimize capitated risk for otherwise healthy individuals.

Medical providers are also starting to realize that they need serious help. Maybe the payors are not yet ready to come back into markets they've already capitated, but other potential soul mates have vested interests in the success or failure of capitated providers. Vendors are one such interested party (see Chapter Seven) but so are associated provider organizations such as home care clinicians, infusion therapy firms, medical instrumentation firms, and home medical equipment distributors. These firms are increasingly bearing subcapitated risk, which means that they suffer economic harm if a medical provider can't manage his or her covered lives appropriately.

There are also medical providers who are rethinking their long-term survival in mature and soon-to-be mature capitated markets. In some cases, these providers are forming MSOs and making themselves attractive for purchase by others. Hence, the nature of their contractual relationships, particularly if they are up for sale, may switch back to a good-risk strategy from a bad-risk strategy, necessitating the cancellation of subcapitation contracts. We are seeing this phenomenon occur in Southern California in mid-1995. At the same time, these groups may start purchasing other groups if their covered lives are too small. The bottom line in all of these machinations, however, is a dissatisfaction with capitation because providers either are unable to manage their managed care business or are unable to manage it well enough; those few providers who are managing capitation well will be in a position of buying up capitated risk in a buyer's market.

Institutional providers are slowly discovering that they are on the equivalent of a sinking ship when it comes to their contractual relationships in mature capitation markets like Southern California. The institutional providers have always believed that HMOs need them. They view the hospital as the hub of a healthcare marketplace and as a necessary contractual entity in the world of capitation. Such basic philosophies are becoming undermined as HMOs decide to start contracting with supergroups that will receive larger capitation payments to cover *both* medical and institutional capitation. Under such a contractual relationship, a medical group—albeit a very large medical group with sufficient market breadth—will be choosing hospitals, not the other way around, and the HMOs will certainly not be choosing the hospitals. This scenario is becoming hospital CEOs' worst nightmare, especially when physicians whom hospitals might not have regarded in the highest esteem suddenly become the ones responsible for the hospitals' livelihood. The hospitals are recognizing very quickly that capitation can force them into relationships with unpopular bedfellows or no relationships at all. These trends are very scary for hospital providers, in that they are being forced out of capitated contractual relationships and into subcapitated relationships.

RATIONING

Without the benefit of knowledge that health plans instinctively have about their enrollees who are not included in capitation contracts, providers know much less—if anything useful—about their capitated enrollees. Because medical providers have no useful information to help them manage their business other than price and cost, it is typically on these criteria that capitated medical practices are managed. In fact, institutional providers have even less information than the gatekeepers. While the gatekeepers might know their enrollees' names, addresses, social security numbers and dates of birth (useful for HMOs but virtually useless for medical and healthcare providers), the institutional provider might know only that there is a defined number of members in a community who must present proof of coverage (e.g., a membership card) before the institution knows that they are included in the hospital's capitation. Thus, the institution has even less information with which to manage capitated business than their medical provider "partners." In either instance, the only commodities left to manage in such flawed systems are price and cost. The only management opportunity for these providers boils down to rationing—and *everybody* loses when healthcare is rationed.

Chapter Five

Minimizing Future Capitation Risk

This chapter will discuss missing elements of capitation as it is currently perceived. These missing elements are currently needed to bring a level of management to the marketplace that does not exist due almost entirely to paradigms that do not embrace the changes capitation represents but merely attempt to retrofit capitation within societal norms resistant to necessary change. The injection of the missing elements into a provider community fixated on price will help providers (1) minimize surprises, (2) improve customer satisfaction and outcomes, (3) take advantage of technological trends and political developments, and (4) retain more capitation dollars as net income without resorting to bad-risk strategies (see Chapter Four) aimed at driving down price with no improvements in operational practices.

Of course, part of the problem is that some 90 percent of providers are unaware that capitation is not a new form of reimbursement and that there are larger implications of capitation beyond price alone. To a lesser degree, another part of the problem is that payors are so fixated on outsourcing via capitation as quickly as possible that they create skeletal provider networks with very limited risk assumption experiences and none of the infrastructures needed to manage capitated business intelligently, responsibly, ethically, and profitably. I see a new trend among payors, however, that may begin to reverse this rush to outsourcing.

NEW COMMITMENTS TO EDUCATION

Payors who went into capitated relationships with providers in the early 1990s are beginning to realize that they outsourced too much. Part of many capitation payments is the requirement of providers to educate their healthy, capitated enrollees about the wellness model. The wellness model assumes that covered individuals will see a physician when they're not sick. The early assumption was that patient education was a part of medical practice and that it should be included in capitation payments. The medical providers, knowingly or unknowingly, accepted capitated relationships with such patient education built in to capitation payments.

The providers were not given the infrastructure to document how much education patients received, how well they retained the education (if they received any), and to what extent such education transformed their healthcare consumption patterns (e.g., how many adult patients brought children to providers when the children were not sick or what portion of patients self-assessed non-emergent medical conditions and sought treatment in physician offices and clinics as opposed to hospital emergency departments). The education needs of providers are larger than patient education alone: They encompass modifying patient behaviors, learning the art of managed care medicine, acquiring tools and guidelines to teach enrollees to manage their own wellness, educating staff members to guide enrollees to manage themselves, helping payors influence enrollees to consume healthcare appropriately, and providing educational resources to subsets of capitated populations who have not yet presented themselves as patients.

ENROLLEE TRANSFORMATIONS

Patient education, as a paradigm, is more appropriate to Disease State Management® than to wellness management (see Chapter Six). By allocating educational resources to *patients,* providers are giving the wrong message to their *enrollees:* If substantial education is available only to patients, incentives are created for enrollees to become patients in order to receive education. Yet the provider loses money incrementally for every patient who presents himself or herself to the provider's office or clinic for treatment. Indeed, healthcare is often considered a *negative want*—people don't normally desire to consume healthcare services. The new paradigm for education must recognize that people need education to stay out of the doctor's office in an appropriate manner and that they would be dissatisfied if they needed to consume healthcare services in order to receive such education. Thus, the new paradigm should seek to provide enrollees with education that helps them avoid unnecessary healthcare consumption. This new paradigm is not concerned with patient education; rather, it is concerned with enrollee education.

The perfect time to transform enrollee consumption patterns is when generally healthy enrollees first join the HMO. At this time, they choose a medical provider to serve as gatekeeper—a choice often influenced by the contracted hospital at which the physician admits the HMO's patients. The HMO then sends the enrollee a confirmation letter, which serves as the first and last communication between the premium payer (the enrollee and his or her dependents) and the premium recipient (the HMO). Sometimes the HMO sends no letter at all, just personalized membership cards with the name, provider number, and physician phone number of the selected gatekeeper(s). In the letter, the payor confirms the "choices" of "gatekeeper" and contracted hospital and indicates that the enrollee should make an appointment with the gatekeeper for virtually free physicals (with perhaps minimal co-payments). This kind of mailing provides no instruction to enrollees about using managed care services appropriately; enrollees can therefore be expected to rely on their previous consumption habits, which are admittedly steeped in the American tradition of the "illness model"—you see a doctor when you're so sick that bedrest and/or over-the-counter drugs no longer provide relief; furthermore, you agree to go to a hospital only when you are deathly ill.

Capitated enrollees can benefit from an alternative approach. Instead of sending a mailing that assumes members will continue previous consumption habits, however inappropriate, the capitated provider should send enrollees a much different kind of letter. The letter might say something like this:

> Welcome to XYZ Medical Group! We're excited that you have selected us to be your gatekeeper as part of your coverage under _____ . Our members are important to us, and we'd like to get to know you so that you're not just some code on a piece of paper.
>
> We are hosting a series of "Open Houses" for families like yours who have recently joined our medical group as part of their HMO coverage. At the Open House you select, we will introduce ourselves, have an opportunity to get to know you and your family, give you a tour of our facilities, have healthcare professionals available to answer any questions you might have, and provide you with delicious refreshments and a thank-you gift. *We will not do any medical tests or perform any medical procedures.* The purpose of this visit is entirely social—for you and your family to meet and feel comfortable with us.
>
> Please indicate below which Open House you and your family feel is most convenient to attend. There is no cost to you and this is entirely outside the covered benefits of your particular HMO. We absorb the cost of these Open Houses as a courtesy to you, our valued members.

Of course, there will be clinical assessments at these open houses, but in a manner that is entirely unobtrusive to the members. Physicians have traditionally overlooked one resource in obtaining clinical assessment data: emergency department nurses, especially triage nurses. These professionals are trained to identify potentially life-threatened individuals on the basis of observation alone. The presence of one triage nurse who silently observes an open house filled with people, or who asks members of the audience to introduce themselves, can help physicians identify individuals who are "walking time bombs": the substance abusers, likely cardiac patients, people with chronic respiratory problems, and so on. Emergency department nurses are the ones who evaluate triage patients in high-pressure, crowded emergency departments; they determine who must be rushed to the trauma room, who should be seen first by the emergency physician(s), and who is well enough to wait until there is a lull. Their typical arsenal rarely involves conversing with patients; rather, careful observation alone is usually sufficient for them to determine the most seriously ill individuals. Their training is perfect for individuals, such as capitated HMO members, who require assessments but have historically stayed away from physicians until they get too sick to ignore a particular problem.

Getting the walking time bombs in to see the physician as early as possible is the first line of attack in transforming enrollees. If the gross assessment is accurate, these individuals might require management as part of a disease state population (see below) instead of as part of a primary care population. Getting to these individuals quickly and initiating aggressive medical management should be a primary consideration; these people will have poor outcomes and survivability under a traditional gatekeeper model (see below).

After the open house, a follow-up questionnaire (by mail or phone) can stratify the remaining enrollees according to those who should be monitored (in person or by phone) and those who really don't need to be monitored within the first three to six months. The questionnaire needs to represent a win–win situation. Beyond providing information *in* to the physician, it needs to provide guiding information *out* to the capitated enrollee and his or her family members. Blue Shield's former "HealthTrack®" product, for example, has nationally maintained statistics regarding some 25 different health status indicators; for a very reasonable fee (historically under $50 per enrollee), this product provides a measurement of the individual's health status per indicator as well as individualized rankings against a statistically valid database. Thus, the questionnaire becomes more than a health information collection tool—it becomes a means by which individual enrollees can manage and be accountable for their own health status.

RIGHTS TO HEALTH OR HEALTHCARE?

The introduction to this book hinted that many of the inequalities associated with capitated managed care stem from the failure of the U.S. government to take an unequivocal stand on how much healthcare should be an American right and to whom such a stand should apply. In reality, the question of the rights of American individuals should focus on how much healthiness education they should receive to *minimize* the amount of healthcare they must have.

I'd like to digress on the latter point. Healthcare is often not a want and, as such, is generally not a discretionary commodity. In other words, if an American family has an extra $150 remaining in its monthly checking account, after all essential expenses are paid, paying for an invigorating colonoscopy (a rectally inserted, cold-metal scope) would be poor competition for a trip to Disneyland. Yet healthcare is often viewed as a negative want and, in the case of disease state populations (see below), a need. The "negative want" concept says that consumption of limited healthcare resources is desirable if it will reduce the need for more serious care later or if it will eliminate the need for certain care that no one truly wants. Thus, a woman might choose a screening mammogram, however uncomfortable and embarrassing the procedure may be, to avoid the later discovery of breast cancer when life-saving or disease-reversing options are no longer viable.

Since 1973, Public Law 93-641 has attempted to portray healthcare as a scarce need that demands governmental control, while at the same time ignoring the market realities of differential provider referral patterns (e.g., a hospital bed is not an undifferentiated commodity; in other words, a bed in a modern regional referral hospital is not the same commodity as a bed in a dilapidated hospital). Many states have since voted to repeal PL 93-641, also called the Health Planning Law, in favor of market-based management of healthcare resources, which differentiates on price, convenience, quality, and outcomes, and no longer just on availability. Now, in many states, the healthcare industry no longer enjoys the protected status afforded it by governmental regulations that involved monopolistic, anticompetitive pricing and availability practices; indeed, hospitals with high-quality patient care teams, low amounts of human error (e.g., medication errors and nosocomial wound infections), and favorable clinical outcomes have better market presence and positioning than their counterparts with PL 93-641 "franchises."

Thus, with a regard to our unalienable rights, I would amend the Declaration of Independence so that the phrase: "life, liberty, and the pursuit of happiness" reads "life, liberty, and the pursuits of happiness and healthiness." The pursuit of healthiness is not really a right in this country, but the entitlement to healthcare is a right for certain individuals (see Introduction) and not a right for most. In other words, I find it unbelievable that the Declaration of Independence entitled people to pursue pleasurable experiences without requiring them to take responsibility for the consequences of such "pleasurable" pursuits as drug use, smoking, overeating, and alcohol consumption. Our historic entitlements, especially for those for whom healthcare is a right, serve to "bail out" such individuals whose excessive pursuits of happiness jeopardize their health. This apparent confusion serves to penalize taxpayers who must compensate the providers for the legitimate excesses of populations entitled to healthcare. The only solution that makes sense to me is that society provide incentives for people to improve their health proactively rather than continue to provide a safety net to individuals who care considerably less about their own healthiness or who are provided insufficient education about healthiness in the first place. This solution extends particularly to the public health sector.

EDUCATING AND MANAGING DISEASE STATE POPULATIONS

The negative want concept of healthcare consumption applies only to healthy populations and to populations at risk who do not already have chronic, life-threatening, or life-altering medical conditions. For those populations with chronic, life-threatening, and/or life-altering disease states, appropriate medical interventions represent opportunities to improve their life situations, cure their conditions, and/or reduce the severity of their disease progressions. In other words, healthcare serves a medical or personal *need*. Examples of such disease states include cancer (oncology); high blood pressure (hypertension); arteriosclerosis (atherosclerosis); cardiac rehabilitation (post–open heart surgery or post–coronary angioplasty); cardiac monitoring (post–heart attack); physical rehabilitation (post–stroke, traumatic brain injured, spinal cord injured, paraplegic); diabetes [Type I (insulin-dependent) and Type II (non-insulin-dependent diabetes mellitus]); HIV+/AIDS; acute burn; and renal-impaired (e.g., dialysis). *Traditional managed care, including traditional gatekeeping, is inapplicable to a population known to be unhealthy.* Because traditional managed care practices, especially traditional capitation strategies, do not work for these populations, a new set of operational and compensation practices must be developed.

Reverse Gatekeeping®

Traditional gatekeeping under capitation presumes that a majority of a population is healthy and in need of primary care, and that the gatekeeper determines to what extent more expensive specialty care is warranted, if at all. Under traditional capitation, the gatekeeping primary care physician (PCP) is paid a capitated rate in return for bearing substantial risk; furthermore, the higher the capitation rate paid to the gatekeeper, the higher the level of risk and/or supported infrastructure such a physician agrees to bear. Under traditional gatekeeping, the PCP receives the lion's share of revenues and the specialists are the beggars.

Under traditional gatekeeping, disease state populations are managed (nonagressively) at the PCP level. When specialty care is needed, often too late to effect substantial reversal or outcomes improvement in the disease state itself, the PCP continues to receive capitation and the specialist is paid on a DFFS or ambulatory case rate basis if the PCP chooses to delegate such care. The specialist's actions must be preapproved by the gatekeeping PCP, at the risk of not receiving compensation. Life-saving interventions that are experimental (and usually very high cost), or not part of the documented mainstream of medical management practice, are rarely authorized by the gatekeeper or the reinsurer for capitated populations even after some high-profile litigation judgments.

The new paradigm for disease state populations should involve high consumption to alter disease states dramatically. Yet historical efforts to change this perspective have been stymied by the financial realities of traditional gatekeeping, especially for disease state populations. The new paradigm involves Reverse Gatekeeping® for these individuals. Reverse Gatekeeping® is, in many respects, the exact opposite of traditional gatekeeping strategies under traditional capitated managed care (see table on the following page).

Comparison of Gatekeeping with Reverse Gatekeeping®

Distinctions	Gatekeeping	Reverse Gatekeeping®
Capitated risk-bearer	Primary care physician	Specialty care physician
Capitation payment basis	Per capita rate, PMPM	Per patient capitated rate
Decision analysis basis	Short-term cost savings	Long-term cost savings
Provider decision scope	Minimalist medical management, minimum approved care	Aggressive medical management, high care consumption
Southern California experience, 1995	Greater than 40%	Less than 1%

In Reverse Gatekeeping® (a registered trademark of Comprehensive Care Corporation), capitation payments made for disease state individuals—per family history and/or medical information obtained by the HMO and/or per claims filed by traditional gatekeepers to the HMO—would accrue to appropriate, risk-bearing, specialty care physicians. (For example, endocrinologists would receive capitation for diabetics, pediatric urological surgeons would receive capitation for Myelomeningocele [spina bifida] children, and immunologists would receive capitation for HIV+ patients.) Such capitation would be calibrated not on the basis of per capita (i.e., per member per month) but on the basis of per disease state patient. Reverse Gatekeeping® capitation payments would be based on a percentage of the fair market value of the annualized costs associated with the average such patient. Actual services under Disease State Management® (a registered trademark of Comprehensive Care Corporation), which the specialist might self-manage or purchase from an MSO or third party, represent an additional responsibility to add to the specialist's capitation (if self-managed), to reduce capitation (if purchased from his or her supplier or MSO), or to pay as subcapitation to others (if purchased from a third party).

Like traditional gatekeeping, physicians providing Reverse Gatekeeping® would bear capitated risk for the medical management (and perhaps institutional management as well) of capitated disease state populations; in so doing, capitation payments would be taken away from the primary care gatekeeper for those specific individuals and recalibrated to an appropriate capitation payment for the appropriate specialty care physician. The specialty care physicians receiving primary capitation or the care of individuals of a specific disease state will maximize their patients' long-term survivability, quality of life, disease-specific adaptation, and long-term outcomes by much higher consumption of fine-tuned diagnostic and aggressive interventional medical (and institutional) care. If current medical patterns of practice are any indication, it is envisioned that such specialists, especially surgeons, would assume the good-risk contracting strategy because it can guarantee a steady flow of patients who truly require their expertise. In addition, current experiences by specialists in traditional gatekeeping have shown them that they are not indispensable to capitated managed care and that stronger PCP retention of populations in need of specialty services, however medically inappropriate, can seriously jeopardize the specialists' ability to stay out of bankruptcy.

Reverse Gatekeeping® is a strategy that helps minimize current and future capitated risk in an area that primary care physicians are unable to manage appropriately. Traditional gatekeeping, whose capitation is based on a per capita formula, is a valid strategy for much less than half the general population. Traditional gatekeeping is inappropriate for the remainder of the general population, including those covered by Medicare. Within that remainder are individuals with known disease states (e.g., individuals who have been diagnosed with a chronic condition such as hypertension), individuals who are at high risk of developing a disease state (e.g., first-degree relatives of those who died from cancer), and individuals who have a chronic condition but do not know it and have not yet been diagnosed (e.g., individuals with diabetes or asymptomatic medical conditions like cancer). Also within the 40 percent remainder are the blind and long-term disabled (including those with end-stage renal disease) who are either covered by, or eligible for, Medicare and whose conditions require major lifestyle adaptations that PCPs are either unqualified to provide or would not likely provide as part of the bad-risk contracting strategy associated with traditional gatekeeping. All of these individuals, including Medicare-eligible seniors who join Medicare Risk plans (an indication that their inclusion within a disease state population is imminent or suspected), should be more appropriately managed via a Disease State Management® strategy that includes Reverse Gatekeeping.® Future decisions must address the one-third of Americans who are severely obese in terms of medical management as healthy populations or as suspect or high-risk disease state populations (such as hypertension and Type II diabetes).

Reverse Gatekeeping® and Disease State Management® Implications

The crossover implications of paying capitation via Reverse Gatekeeping^{SM} while utilizing a Disease State Management® strategy involve giving specialty physicians incentives to manage their covered disease lives more aggressively in the earlier stages of the disease. This strategy would create the following win–win goals both for payors eager to market the successes of their contracted providers at improving health and for unhealthy individuals

- To reduce the probability of complicating conditions (which cost the risk-bearer more money).
- To introduce a "front-loading" aspect to capitation that reduces the liability for higher infirmity later in a patient's disease progression.
- To improve earlier disease adaptation, which would be more cost advantageous than continuing to subsidize individuals who have not adapted to their condition (e.g., weaning ventilator-dependent paraplegics).
- To improve long-term outcomes at lower overall cost (e.g., keeping age-onset diabetics from requiring insulin and/or oral hypoglycemics—at recurring, high, pharmacy and consumables expense—thereby being managed better on diet and exercise alone).

Primary care physicians to whom traditional gatekeeping has been delegated and who now receive capitation for disease state populations are not likely to invest financial resources in these, or most any, covered lives. The reason for this lack of investment is not that they are bad physicians or that they don't care about practicing good, managed care medicine. The reason is that traditional gatekeeping precludes the necessity to make *medical* decisions. **Traditional gatekeeping substitutes *financial* decision making for actual medical decisions.**

PCPs who practice traditional gatekeeping within a medical group, a staff-model HMO, or an MCO that utilizes IPAs are given an incentive to reduce consumption of expensive diagnostic and therapeutic procedures. While this strategy is important in removing wasteful practices associated with managing nonchronic patient populations (e.g., fine-tuning diagnostic practices to order specific lab tests to confirm a hypothesized medical condition rather than to order bundled, "shotgun" lab tests to formulate hypothetical diagnoses in the absence of a reliable history and physical exam and/or very low-cost diagnostics), it is highly inappropriate for diagnosing higher-cost acute or chronic medical conditions that are undefinitive without the more expensive diagnostic procedures.

For example, a colorectal surgeon specializing in treating prostate cancer, who might receive Reverse Gatekeeping® capitation for both victims of prostate cancer and their sons, would readily perform periodic, screening colonoscopies on the victims' sons, even if they are so far asymptomatic. By contrast, a medical group, which includes surgeons and pediatricians, receiving full-risk medical capitation on either a good-risk or a bad-risk basis, might perform screening colonoscopies only on those who are symptomatic of prostate cancer and who "failed" a physician's touch-test during a physical examination (which, by such action, would exclude the vast majority of individuals who are the "silent victims" of prostate cancer). Even though the cost of a screening colonoscopy is $200 to $300, the gatekeeper will typically weigh the expected benefit of the test against the known cost; it is highly unlikely, in this case, that asymptomatic young men—even if their fathers have contracted prostate cancer—would receive screening colonoscopies before the age of 50.

In the above discussion, I am raising two points:

1. Who bears the risk for early detection? If specialists bear the risk for victims and high-risk populations (including first-degree relatives of victims, however asymptomatic), it shouldn't matter to primary care physicians how the risk-bearers choose to self-manage that risk.

2. Specialty physicians bearing capitated risk should not be forced to behave like primary care physicians in managing that risk.

Giving specialists subcapitation according to market pricing, as inherent in full-risk medical capitation, does not empower them to behave as specialists in managing risk. Part of the reason is that specialists are trained to manage patients with specific conditions (and only those conditions), not to manage a general population where individuals with the specific condition are not pre-identified by the subcapitating physician (and assumed not to exist) and where the total sample of individuals who might have such a condition represents a relatively small percentage of individuals in the population (i.e., finding needles in a haystack). This practice is convenient for a full-risk medical group or IPA, a PCP gatekeeper, or an MCO practicing on a community-wide basis; it is highly inappropriate for specialists intent on managing individual patients with specialized medical conditions.

Specialty subcapitation under traditional managed care models forces specialists into bad-risk contracting strategies, all aimed at furthering an agenda based on rationing; the market prices of specialty subcapitation (e.g., 18 to 25 cents PMPM for neurology subcapitation) require either finding a lower-bidding specialist (buying in to the bad-risk approach) for the same lives or agreeing to a dilution of earnings by providing real specialty care to diagnosed individuals. Just as it's unfair to expect PCPs to subsidize capitation rates to provide medical care as part of a good-risk contracting strategy, it is inappropriate to expect specialty care physicians to make similar financial sacrifices. The conclusion I've reached is that this new system of capitated managed care is needed to integrate different health management strategies with the gatekeeper concept.

INFORMATION SUPERHIGHWAY IMPLICATIONS

The term *information superhighway* has been abused more often than it has been used appropriately. The purpose of its inclusion in this book is to point out the implications of the existence of the information super-highway for minimizing capitation risks. A parallel purpose is to recognize current opportunities related to capitated managed care in mature markets.

Many of the positive implications of managing capitation business relate to the key developments in the creation of the information super-highway. Unlike many of my colleagues, I do not consider the information superhighway to be synonymous with the Internet; rather, the term represents a confluence of technological advancements and a resultant change in society relative to the new capabilities. In this regard, I consider the Internet as a tool for improving individuals' access to greater stores of diverse information, rather than as a virtual theme park for increasingly computer-literate thrillseekers. The increasing proliferation of satellite-based technologies will improve such access as well.

One of the most significant improvements in technological capabilities, I feel, is the rapid proliferation of fiber optics, particularly in telecommunications cabling. One of the first fiber-optic hubs in American telecommunications sits under Southern California's Los Angeles International Airport in preparation for the 1984 Summer Olympics there. The hub was created to boost media coverage of the Los Angeles Olympics, particularly to allow journalists covering Olympic events instantaneous access to their editors in other parts of the world.

Unfortunately, integrated networks of increasingly capitated providers in Southern California are not taking advantage of fiber-optic technologies, which have been more advanced in this market than elsewhere in America for nearly a decade. These integrated networks are not utilizing fiber optics to share electronic medical records (EMR) among their providers; in fact, less than 5 percent of Southern California's providers' practices (medical and/or hospital) have moved to electronic patient records as an alternative to paper-based records. Despite the 1994 Northridge (actually the Reseda) earthquake, when hundreds of physician offices lost tens of thousands of patient records as a result of earthquake and/or water damage, almost none have made the switch to EMR. In the case of this technology, capitated providers have remained either skeptical or too cost conscious to prepare for the next major earthquake by making the transition to EMR and to take advantage of fiber optics in sharing records within integrated networks.

What I consider a key development, one many might consider surprising, was the decision by the Health Care Financing Administration in the middle of 1992 to create delays in paying Medicare claims, starting in January 1993, for providers who did not utilize electronic billing. Starting in January 1993, providers who submitted paper-based claims experienced a minimum two-week delay in getting their Medicare claims paid; by contrast, providers submitting claims via modem received their money within two to three days. That hardware and software prices were so low at the time (under $500 for a no-frills personal computer, $50 for a 2400-baud modem, and $15 for the software packet purchased from the provider's fiscal intermediary) hastened many providers to move to the computer age and to electronic billing. With the addition of electronic data interchange (EDI) technology about a year later, which allowed for the debiting and crediting of providers' bank accounts electronically in response to electronically billed claims, providers had truly paperless patient accounting systems, but paper-based everything else. Medicare's incentives to providers to join the electronic computer age represented a tremendous boost to their ability to utilize resources that were being created for the eventual information superhighway, even though the promise remains largely unrealized.

Another major technological development leading to the creation of the information superhighway was the introduction of asynchronous transfer mode (ATM) technology. ATM represented a transmission protocol that allows for rapid, two-way sharing of voluminous information. Examples of healthcare applications that can benefit from this technology include telemedicine (e.g., teleradiology), satellite-based medicine, the ability to transmit two-way digital cable and HDTV over telephone wires (which are becoming increasingly fiber-optic), and the ability to allow for real-time, bidirectional communications between providers sharing the same information (including video).

Very few medical providers have installed even the most basic packet communication systems to share electronic mail, voice mail, digitized radiographic images, digitized tracings (e.g., fetal heart monitor tracings for obstetricians, Holter or EKG monitor tracings for cardiologists, and EEG tracings for neurologists), digitized video, and/or digitized video stills (photographs). All of these media are available at relatively low cost in mid-1995, and have been available to physicians who would have purchased them for at least the last three years. Communication programs that marry these and an increasing array of newer capabilities (such as automated patient and surgical scheduling modules) have been available for over five years; in many cases, MCOs eager to facilitate meaningful provider communications in a cost-effective manner have been willing to subsidize such technologies for their loyal physicians.

Perhaps the most important implication of the technological advances related to the information superhighway is represented by the increasing transformation of healthcare consumers themselves. As a result of the 1994 Christmas gift-giving season, which was the strongest holiday season over the previous three years, the low price and streamlined distribution channels of personal computers had a tremendous effect. A recent study of Americans' gift purchases from the 1994 holiday season reveals that approximately half of American households with incomes above $40,000 have personal computers, and 25 percent of households with incomes below $20,000 have PCs as well.

The implications of the computerization of America are quite startling. Television and radio broadcasters seized the opportunity of creating media forums for customers of commercial online services (such as Microsoft Access, America Online, Prodigy, and CompuServe); businesses began catering to computerized customers by creating artistically appealing "Home Pages" on Internet's World Wide Web; and entrepreneurial individuals created their own "Home Pages" as a new distribution channel with far greater consumer reach and frequency than conventional promotional tactics—and at far less expense. In effect, Baby Boomers could now be marketed via modem. The intermarriage of telephone, computer, and cable television capabilities by single vendors is enhancing the convenience of such offerings to increasingly receptive consumers. Capabilities we can expect within the next year include wellness-based cable-TV programming customized by providers to specific individuals, who can view such programming on either their TV sets or their interconnected computer monitors and can respond back.

A concurrent development related to the half of middle-class American households with computers is that the computers they purchased increasingly have CD-ROM, always a powerful technology but only recently fast enough and inexpensive enough to be in demand by consumers. While various computer-assisted, medical diagnosis products (also known as "doc-in-the-box" software) have been available for PCs over the last 10 years, the interface was text-based, clunky, and unappealing to most consumers. Today's software packages, including co-branding by prestigious hospitals such as the Mayo Clinic and Johns Hopkins University, utilize CD-ROM technology and are bundled by manufacturers with the purchase of the unit itself.

The implication of consumers, particularly young families and single parents, having CD-ROM-based medical diagnosis software includes the overnight sophistication of healthcare consumers. Some of the software is reasonably accurate in diagnosing a child's likely condition, and parents using it are given very specific questions that, when asked of their human providers, will give them the information they need to know in a way that best protects them against human error or judgment lapses. How many providers, rather than continuing to fight this technology, are encouraging their patients to use it and to take responsibility for their own health status and the health status of their family? Isn't this end the *purpose* of capitated managed care? The truly unbelievable part is that the cost of owning such software is relatively low, and that enlightened providers could negotiate volume discounts with the software publishers so that the technology would cost even less to implement.

THE PRICE OF RISK MINIMIZATION

This chapter recognizes the implications of education, gatekeeping (both traditional and Reverse Gatekeeping®), and technology as strategies to minimize current risks associated with capitated managed care. The message I wish to convey is that many of these risk-minimization strategies involve little more than changing a paradigm. Gatekeeping was never intended to be an exact, self-limiting science. The inventors of gatekeeping had to have known that the market would improve the concept to take better care of larger segments of individuals incorporated within capitated managed care. Gatekeeping, like capitation, represents a set of management strategies and not a self-limiting contractual strategy. Just as capitation is not limited to fixing payments to providers, so too is gatekeeping more than an implement of cost control and service rationing. Gatekeeping involves tending the gate appropriately, whether for increased consumptive needs by disease state populations or for less wasteful practices that PCPs should be using in employing the art of managed care medicine. In addition, providers are the last in the current marketplace to take full advantage of computerization and technological advances that their capitated enrollees *expect* to be utilized.

Chapter Six

Maximizing Opportunities with Capitation Management

This chapter will discuss critical success strategies for improving the management of capitated individuals, using both traditional and Reverse Gatekeeping® techniques. The chapter will provide measurable objectives to allow capitated enrollees to take responsibility for their own health status—the goal of *true* capitation in general—whether they are part of wellness-based or disease-state populations. Much of the promise of this chapter will be for relatively immature capitated markets, which are interested in creating capitated business the "right way" rather than replicating the mistakes of mature capitation markets like Southern California. It is unrealistic to assume that mature capitation markets can unlearn their bad habits and rewrite their history; the future truly belongs to those communities that are looking for the gold standards of creating and managing capitation business, a set of standards that have never really existed until now.

PROVIDER DEFINITIONS RELATED TO CAPITATION MANAGEMENT

In my personal dictionary, the definition of capitation management goes along with my new definition of capitation in that it relates to the outsourcing of health management and not to the manner in which providers are paid. Many MCOs take the provider payment approach, referring to capitation management as the set of cost management strategies to coax more revenue retention from capitation payments. Yet it is precisely this financial-only perspective to capitation that has over-focused providers and consumers on the compensation aspects and led to widespread rationing of healthcare consumption. Without a strategy-oriented definition of capitation (see the sports-playing example in Chapter Two), providers and managers are left to deal with the aspects of capitation with which they are comfortable; hence, their definitions of capitation are compensation-driven and their capitation management strategies are financially driven from the standpoint of maximizing compensation.

In contrast, and as a consequence, my definition of the term *capitation management* is as follows:

> Capitation management is a set of proactive strategies geared to enhance the health and/or wellness of covered lives toward the goal of preparing enrollees and their families to take responsibility for their own health status.

I believe that providers, especially PCPs, would prefer to manage health and wellness instead of being so cost- and nonconsumption-driven that they easily lose sight of why they chose to be primary care physicians. They frequently perceive that capitation is a necessary evil they must embrace to remain competitive in a mature capitation market. Yet I believe that capitation itself is not evil unless a provider adopts a bad-risk contracting strategy, which requires a negative perspective in order to be successful at capitation. As I discussed at greater length in Chapter Four, there are very few aspects of the bad-risk contracting strategy from either the medical provider, institutional provider, or consumer standpoint that can point to success; it is largely a *failed strategy* that creates enmity among providers and distrust and fear in the eyes of consumers. A system that relies even 25 percent on providers who practice a bad-risk strategy in "managing" their capitation business reflects a market that has no real system for managing care that provides for measurable improvements in health status.

STRATEGIES CONTRIBUTING TO THE FAILURE OF CAPITATION

Before we can talk about winning strategies that guarantee success, I think it's time to evaluate candidly the set of losing strategies that guarantee the failure of capitation markets. I believe that markets contemplating a move to capitation should understand what doesn't work, in the hopes that the world can learn from our mistakes in Southern California and not blindly replicate our failures. I see the seeds of failure now being sown in markets, most notably in America's southern and mid-atlantic states, where financial and contracting managers from Southern California are being imported strictly on their ability to generate and preserve capitation contracts that depend on rationing and managing cost; and yet, these managers have no real track records in enhancing community health and improving and managing individual members' health status.

The Element of Surprise

The key complaint of providers in considering a move to capitation is the element of surprise. If no information is given to providers to help them understand the medical and institutional needs of the population for whom they are capitated, they will always be surprised. Their surprise will have a steep price for them if their medical or institutional needs are surprisingly high (yet if no information is given to determine which needs are at very high cost and which needs are at a relatively affordable cost, every need will be considered unaffordable). Their surprise will be compounded if their assumptions about the health status and health needs of their capitated population are very far off base. Yet, again, when capitated providers are given no information and no wherewithal for self-generating information as to what the inherent health statuses and inherent health needs are for their capitated population, they will have no basis for determining if their assumptions are true or false.

Over time, such providers will come to realize that the only thing they can count on is that they will be surprised. These providers create strategies so that they will be surprised less often, not by seeking out hidden sources of necessary information to prevent surprises but by restricting access to their capitated populace—who will only surprise them anyway. Hence, the result is a vicious cycle of rationing based on denial. The tragedy is that less than 1 percent of all capitated providers in Southern California have any useful information for all of their capitated population (whether or not those people have been prior patients of a physician or hospital that has received capitation for their health management).

How Payors Handle Surprises

The providers who receive full-risk medical or full-risk institutional capitation are paid by a payor who chooses capitation as a means of outsourcing its own responsibility for health management of defined populations. While most capitation-based systems are structured so that all providers will be surprised by the patients who walk through their doors, the payors themselves are less comfortable with the element of surprise than the providers to whom capitation is offered. The payors collect a great deal of information about self-employed applicants for HMO coverage as well as from small-employee companies with two to five covered individuals—the vast majority of businesses in the United States. It is true that limited health and medical information is obtained about individual employees and their families within medium and large companies; hence, payors determine what information they give capitated providers based on what information they have from the most restricted sources (e.g., very large employers and ERISA [Employee Retirement Income Security Act of 1974, pursuant to Public Law 93-406] benefit plans). Generally, the information payors give to their capitated providers (namely, those providers contracted for full medical or institutional risk directly by the payor) comprises all of the following:

1. Names of employee and dependents.
2. Social security numbers of employee and dependents.
3. Employee's address.
4. Dates of birth of employee and dependents.

Obviously, the foregoing information is appropriate for the payor to give providers for all covered lives, but these represent merely pieces of data that providers can't really use as a substitute for the information they really need: inherent health status and medical/institutional health needs of their covered lives. They need better information about their capitated responsibilities, not just relatively useless data that the payor can conveniently provide. However, are there things the providers should infer about the kind of data payors give them?

Perhaps providers should start putting themselves in the payors' shoes and learn more about the payor industry itself, so that they can understand the data given to them within the proper context. *Payors are not providers.* Perhaps this statement seems obvious, but it is a fact lost on many a provider. Providers originate from the medical, nursing, allied health, and healthcare management industries. Payors originate from the insurance industry. Providers and payors behave like members of their own industries.

As mentioned in Chapter Two, when providers are faced with a challenge they can't control (e.g., managing capitated populations without meaningful information or responding to changes in the way payors reimburse providers on DFFS), they create solutions to help them be incrementally successful—for example, restricting access to capitated populations via shortened hours of operation, fewer phone lines, more dead-end voice mail installations, and fewer physicians; or creating unbundled billing and/or upcoding strategies to coax more reimbursement out of each procedure performed.

By contrast, when payors are faced with a challenge they can't control, they run away. This strategy is the same positioning strategy used by other members of the insurance industry. This escapist strategy explains why physicians are hard-pressed to find professional liability insurance anymore, why professional service organizations are challenged to find directors and officers liability insurance, why Southern California residents can no longer find affordable (or even unaffordable) earthquake insurance, and why so few insurance carriers continue to write affordable indemnity-based health insurance. When the loss ratios get too high, the payors are challenged to buy affordable underwriting. If the price of underwriting is too high to cover an insurance product, they either increase the price of the product (in markets where there is an elasticity of price) or cancel the policies of customers who are covered by the product.

One of the strategies insurance companies use to increase the price of an insurance product in markets where there is an elasticity of price is a procedure called *redlining*. The term *redlining* is often used in the automobile insurance industry, where residents of one zip code pay more for the same or similar coverage than residents of a zip code with lower or less expensive loss experience. Redlining also leads to some form of community ratings, where the insurance companies begin to rate the various communities within a given market according to numbers of filed claims, the losses associated with those claims, and their own profit margins associated with those communities. Thus, redlining forms a base strategy for repricing premiums, recalibrating profit margins, and encouraging or discouraging sales within a given community.

Within the healthcare industry, payors' roots in insurance industry techniques like redlining have tremendous implications for providers. Redlining defines which communities within a given market have stronger correlations with high-dollar medical losses and undesirable medical risk. While many state governments have clamped down on premiums that are restricted or overpriced due to redlining practices, the practices by payors with regard to capitation are quite insidious because the redlining strategies are transparent to the public and to regulators.

The impact of redlining on capitation pricing really boils down to a strictly financial decision. Since capitation represents outsourcing by the payor to providers for the health management of defined populations, the payor has the responsibility of determining for which defined populations it will apply capitated pricing. The provider is wrong to assume that all customers of a payor, especially within an immature capitation market, are included within capitation-based pricing because capitation represents a fixed accounts payable responsibility to the payor. Quite simply, the payor chooses which populations to self-manage through reimbursement-based pricing (including case pricing, DFFS, and UCR) and which to outsource via capitation. If you haven't already guessed, the redlining technique is the one most often used by payors as a decision criterion in determining exactly which defined populations are to be sold to providers as a fixed accounts payable—as part of capitated pricing.

The implications of the use of redlining in the offering of defined populations by payors for capitated pricing are quite substantial. Using the redlining technique and simple financial logic, it is likely that the payor will continue to self-manage defined populations with low medical loss ratios, with acceptably low numbers of filed medical or hospitalization claims, and/or with relatively low-cost claims experience. It is also likely that the payor will first offer to capitation the defined populations with the highest loss ratios, with the worst claims experience, and with the most adverse health status risks (e.g., high-crime, high-violence inner-city and outlying areas, and markets with high concentrations of populations most at risk for HIV+/AIDS).

Until the market matures quite substantially to the point that the payor is ready to move all, or substantially all, of its healthcare customers to capitated contracts and get out of the healthcare management/adjudication business within that defined market, the payor will continue to self-manage the lowest-cost populations. From the providers' standpoint, this means that the business offered to them on a capitated basis will be the book of business that the payor chooses not to self-manage. In other words, the business they will be buying includes overly high utilizers of medical and/or institutional healthcare services, and/or those inherently too risky for the payor to continue to self-manage. The corollary to this reality, which few providers are ready to realize, is that the normal incidence and prevalence rates of major diseases do not generally apply in the purchase of capitated risk. Yet providers have always assumed that they can insulate themselves from such risk by purchasing large enough populations of capitated members. This capitation strategy, which ignores the insurance industry realities associated with redlining practices, can serve to *increase* adverse risk exposure rather than decrease it.

I consider it safe to say that payors are not telling providers within immature capitated markets *why* the capitated populations are for sale. In addition, payors give scant information to providers for two reasons: (1) the data provided represent most of what payors genuinely know about *all* of their enrollees; and (2) payors want the data to be of very little use in helping providers understand the populations they are buying. This limitation of disclosure reflects a profit-oriented, adversarial relationship on the part of payors. If providers understood more of what they are buying from payors at the time of sale, they might have some inkling that they are buying "defective merchandise." The old Latin adage "caveat emptor" (let the buyer beware) is especially appropriate. Providers need to understand some of the payor's selling motivations to truly understand what they are buying. Providers also need to reduce their naiveté and develop strategies to defend against payors who are looking for buyers of capitated populations.

Differential Payor Risk Assumption

Providers should try to avoid jumping right into high stop-loss-level capitation arrangements without some experience. The strategy involves what is called *risk bands* or *risk corridors*. The strategy is particularly appropriate for providers with little to no prior capitation experience and is a strategy MCOs are willing to exercise in transitioning desirable providers toward assuming full capitation risk on a gradual basis. Risk banding involves limiting the capitation rate to a maximum cap tied to a predicted usage of services, with current market ranges for caps between 2 and 5 percent. Utilization above the cap is paid by the MCO according to a set rate, a discounted fee-for-service, or an additional capitation rate; it is similar to the way Medicare DRGs compensate: a defined DRG rate for a defined case mix with additional compensation for outliers. Under risk banding, capitation is structured for a defined mix or acuity of patients and excludes high usage or outlier cases such as HIV+/AIDS, oncology, high-acuity pediatrics, and rehabilitation patients. Providers should also work with the MCO's information systems department to collect data on all patients managed and begin benchmarking techniques to define best practices by diagnosis while developing models for predicting utilization. These predictive and modeling applications are critical tools for capitation management.

Another differential payor risk assumption technique involves risk sharing. The parties to a risk-sharing approach to capitation agree to a below-market rate for the desired services and design a reward system, such as a percentage of savings to their relationship by substituting refinements to diagnostic structures for additional consumption of hospital services, such as the benefit of reduced exploratory surgeries when certain examinations are performed first. The parties will enjoy greater reward for successes than for being paid at full market rates. The parties evaluate their risk and reward system on an ongoing basis to ensure that both of them benefit from the arrangement, and they experiment with other risk-sharing arrangements to determine the most advantageous trade-offs between risk and reward.

Finally, I'd like to describe how medical providers use capitation as a means for managing their business better. How medical providers manage their practices has to do with the proportion of capitation business on which their operation is dependent. A capitation penetration rate of 15 percent or less allows providers to dabble freely, provided they are in immature or developing capitation markets. They can expand or reduce the amount of capitated business relatively freely without serious repercussions to their core business.

A capitation penetration of 15 to 45 percent means that the provider is quite serious about being successful in capitation. At the higher end of this range, capitation is one of the organization's top three payor classes. A decision by a payor or a subcapitating provider organization not to renew a capitation contract by the provider with 15 to 45 percent penetration could jeopardize a significant portion of the business. Providers within this range who are participating in point-of-service plans, whereby they are part of an HMO panel on a temporary basis (see Chapter Two), are hurt most if the HMO removes the provider from the panel or does not renew the POS offer because the loss of the business, coupled with the loss of base business that the capitation business replaced, has an additive impact on the provider's practice. Finally, providers with this amount of capitated business are generally looking to capitation as their primary source of referrals and should begin preparing for full capitation.

A penetration over 45 percent means that half or more of the provider's business is dependent on capitation. This amount of capitation is what I call full capitation in that providers should begin setting their infrastructure to manage in line with capitated business. Provider groups in the upper end of this range, with a capitation penetration of 75 percent or more, treat noncapitated business as the anomaly and capitation as the standard.

In treating capitation as the standard for a provider organization's infrastructure, the providers start viewing their revenues as fixed PMPMs (per Patient per Month for providers involved in Reverse Gatekeeping®) and begin looking at their fixed and variable operating expenses as PMPM offsets. In other words, the providers receiving PMPM (fixed) revenues attempt to convert all of their operating expenses to fixed by budgeting each line item according to its PMPM effect on PMPM revenues. In this manner, budgeting becomes very simple: PMPM revenues minus PMPM expenses equals PMPM profit. Evaluating PMPM expenses can be as simple as taking predictive monthly expenses divided by the provider's covered lives to yield a PMPM equivalent. On a tougher level, providers start looking to their vendors to go at risk by charging PMPM prices for goods and services previously priced on the basis of consumption; this transformation of vendors to ones who look to PMPM pricing involves what I call vendor capitation (see Chapter Seven).

CRITICAL SUCCESS STRATEGIES FOR CAPITATION MANAGEMENT

The critical success strategies that a provider should be taking for ensuring his or her success at managing capitation business relate to the following objectives:

1. Identify reality and take stock of actual information.
2. Transform enrollee behavior to one that supports the wellness model.
3. Encourage and support enrollees' health improvement efforts.
4. Track and document all instances of consumption, including behaviors that both drive and restrain enrollee consumption.
5. Use behavior modification to encourage enrollees to be and remain successful at health and/or wellness improvement.
6. Generate a consistent feedback loop between enrollees and providers.

Identifying Reality

As previously mentioned with regard to redlining, providers are hesitant to change their inherent assumptions that payors are selling normal distributions and that more volume minimizes inherent risk. Even though the reality is that redlining practices in immature capitation markets tempt payors to sell populations that are either unmanageable or are not worth the payor's continuing to self-manage, providers do not ask informed questions, do not understand why payors outsource, and do not realize that the payors know more about the populations they're selling than the amount of information provided would suggest. If asked, payors should be able to divulge the medical loss ratios of the population being sold to capitation—not necessarily on an individualized basis, but certainly on the basis of community ratings.

Because the deck is stacked against novice providers who have no risk-banding experience prior to contracting for capitated business, the provider needs to know what's real. If a provider group is capitated for 10,000 individuals, the provider needs to know the reality concerning each and every member for whom it is capitated, rather than falsely projecting populations at risk on the basis of incidence and prevalence rates that do not apply for defined groups of individuals sold under capitation. Often the payor provides no assistance in helping the provider learn about each and every person for whom he or she is capitated, neither in manpower, computer, nor telephonic support. These providers need to learn as much about their population, and as quickly and effectively as possible, *before* the patients surprise their caregivers by showing up in offices and clinics with serious at-risk, acute, and chronic medical conditions.

The use of the Reverse Gatekeeper® approach (see Chapter Five) for populations with serious acute and chronic medical conditions represents an opportunity to save PCPs from becoming very surprised that they are being asked to manage disease state populations for capitated pricing that presumes the populations are healthy or in need of relatively low levels of services. It is on this premise that commercial capitation rates are founded, and upon which justification that such per capita pricing is set. Payors probably never intended to bundle Disease State Management® with wellness management, because they represent two completely different systems of managing risk. The offering of specialty subcapitation as part of a bad-risk contracting strategy is indeed odious because specialists are not given the right mix of resources to practice their craft. The solution, of course, is to allow for specialists to assume Reverse Gatekeeping® risk for disease state populations (involving the reduction of PMPM for specific individuals reassigned to a disease state population by the payor) and to allow PCPs to continue to assume traditional gatekeeping risk for wellness-based (non–disease state) populations.

Transforming Enrollee Behavior

Since the goal of capitation is to get enrollees to take responsibility for their own health status and that of their families, a critical intervening step is to start transforming enrollee behavior. A critical area of this transformation has to do with attitudes between enrollee and caregiver.

As stated earlier, the role of the provider changes dramatically under capitation in that the physician is compensated to assume outsourced health management on behalf of the payor or subcapitator. At the same time, any consumptive incident, and especially a consumptive incident that requires the filing of a claim, works against a provider's ability to be financially successful. Just as the onus for providing capitation management in new ways falls on the provider who desires to maximize revenue retention under capitation, so too is there a concomitant shift in consumer attitudes toward providers.

Consumers need to be sensitized to the new role of the provider under capitation. The trick is not to force consumers to change by virtue of the requirements of capitation because capitation is negotiated in a manner that is hidden from consumers. Rather, the strategy involves a gradual easing of the consumer into a new relationship with providers, one that is user-friendly, satisfaction-driven, and committed to helping consumers lead healthier and less stressful lives. The jackhammer approach that providers and their clinical and nonclinical staffs have been using for the last few years, especially in the wake of the need for cost-cutting and economies of scale that have recently crept into physician offices, works against a kinder and gentler approach.

Encouraging Enrollee Efforts toward Health Management

The basic marketing approach I am suggesting in summarizing this kinder and gentler relationship between enrollees and providers involves basic guest relations. People are motivated when they are respected.

Rather than affording their patients a modicum of respect, certainly more so than in a typical seller-customer approach, many physicians have tried to force their patients to respect them with no reciprocity. The time for soothing providers' egos is past. It is time to use capitation as an opportunity for 1990s providers to reestablish the doctor–patient relationship they lost in the 1980s. This time, however, the need is not for a "god versus mortal" relationship but for one that commands mutual respect.

Capitated providers should come to respect their enrollees' efforts and demonstrated abilities to improve their health and that of their family. The transformation of enrollee behavior can't really occur until physicians change their paradigms of practice. Punitive posturing does not work with enrollees, especially when the desired output is transformed behavior. I can't be clear enough on this concept: **People must be positively motivated to change, not punished** (itself a negative form of motivation) **for not changing.** The implications for enrollee relations and patient relationships are profound. Physicians should refrain from making negative comments or chastisements to patients who are overweight, who smoke, who consume alcohol, or who practice other unhealthy lifestyles. The concept is similar to that involved with spanking a child: Even though a parent might displace some hostility or frustration in the process, the child learns to fear the parent and to give the parent "no bad news." Patients have learned to regard their physicians in the same manner, to the detriment of frank and open dialogue and to the loss of a relationship built on mutual respect and admiration.

Here's an example of a paradigm shift: Would it be so terrible for a physician to offer a $1,000 cash bonus each year to every member who remains within 20 percent of his or her ideal body weight? Remember, in order to claim the cash, members have to come to the physician, when they're not sick, to be measured for both height and weight to determine an ideal weight as well as corridors for optimal weight management (an example of providing members with information to help them manage themselves), and to *choose voluntarily* to see a physician to monitor their weight control progress and claim a reward. Also, in a system that includes Disease State Management® as a parallel managed care system, enrollees within 20% of ideal body weight guarantee retention of a PCP's market share! If members do not return to the physician after a year of being assessed, the physician should infer that they are tracking their weight and that they did not do well enough to claim the prize. Rather than do nothing until they come in—the old paradigm—the enlightened physician should initiate a call to monitor their progress and assess whether their health status has worsened to the degree that an in-person examination might be required. In other words, the physician assists enrollees in providing their own preventive maintenance, similar to the care used in maintaining machines and valued possessions. The provider needs to teach enrollees that their body is one such valued possession and to offer them incentives to do the right things rather than punish them for lapses in judgment.

Here's another paradigm shift: Payors and MCOs should be marketing their associations with enterprises that support enrollee transformational behavior. Have payors or MCOs ever approached the Pritikin organization for co-branding products that can be cross-promoted? Might this organization be looking for payors and MCOs that support their objectives, to whom they could refer their members? Why not add a payor's logo to the labels of Pritikin products to build an association in the minds of consumers that such a payor is supportive of the organization's efforts to reduce fat in Americans' diets and to promote a healthy lifestyle? These payors and MCOs do not have to look far beyond the Pritikin organization to support this new paradigm. Most every food manufacturer is adding low- and non-fat product lines to their offerings that could be co-supported by manufacturers, payors, and key providers. The message that they should be conveying is the same, whether to existing members or to future members.

Part of this enrollee transformation involves transforming enrollee maturity. Saying that the goal of capitation is to allow enrollees to take responsibility for their health status is one thing, but getting them ready to accept responsibility for their health status is quite another. Members of the provider community have been treating their patients and capitated enrollees as children, similar to a parent repeatedly telling a toddler the word *no*. Just as it is difficult for a parent to gently let go as their children become teenagers, it is this exact technique that providers should be using for their capitated enrollees. We need to teach people about the "owner's manual" for their own bodies because this approach teaches the cause–effect relationship between lifestyles and lifestyle-directed behaviors on health status.

Providers can no longer afford to condone their capitated enrollees' child-like behavior when it comes to health status management. They need to understand that there is a cause–effect relationship between smoking and cancer, between unhealthy eating plus sedimentary lifestyle and obesity, between the amount of fat in one's diet and cardiovascular disease, and so on. The way the relationship is presented today is something even children can recite: "Don't smoke! Just say no to drugs! Don't overeat! Fat is ugly! Smoking is for buttheads!"

Rather than emphasizing the negative or punitive aspects of these cause–effect relationships, providers should begin using the new paradigm. Many people are unaware, for example, of the cause–effect relationship that adding fiber to one's diet has on diabetes, or how the addition of antioxidant foods and cruciferous vegetables can lower one's risk of developing certain types of cancer, or how one can enjoy the health benefits of vitamin C if they can't tolerate the acidity of citrus fruits, or how many high-quality years a smoker can add to one's life by quitting smoking today. The relationship between lifestyle and health status is the same, whether couched in negative or positive terms. The difference, really, is how effective the approach is in influencing positive changes in lifestyle and the extent to which such changes improve people's ability to monitor, and make adjustments to, the health status of themselves and their family.

The way these and other guided relationships between capitated enrollee and provider are articulated have value beyond the content alone. The capitated enrollees begin to understand that the provider truly respects them and that the advice is given not to soothe an ego but to imbue them with the knowledge they need in order to understand their own bodies and to develop health management strategies for themselves and their families. Americans are ready to take control of their lives, and the full extent of media, computer, and educational resources is available to guide them. They just need a well-meaning gesture that indicates that the provider is their advocate, their coach, their maintenance technician, and their friend. Providers need to restrain themselves from pushing others; rather, they should demonstrate a willingness to offer incentives and reward those who successfully push themselves. In this manner, a true transformation of enrollee behavior can begin to occur.

Tracking and Documenting Consumptive Incidents and Behaviors

Most providers now document the healthcare consumption demanded by their capitated enrollees. That's the good news. The bad news is that they typically document the wrong things, they don't document the right things, and they throw away the most valuable data of all: documentation that could be used to predict ambulatory outcomes and track behaviors that could lead to improved management of health status. What is often documented are cross-sectional incidents of consumption in the form of a claim;

to most providers, the purpose of a claim is to document what the payor determines needs to be documented, all for the sole purpose of getting paid. What is often undocumented are the longitudinal approaches that could be taken with claims to observe trends and track behavior. What is often thrown away are valuable data in the temporary possession of the provider (or even more temporarily in the provider's head) that, while perhaps important for creating ambulatory outcomes, are not required when submitting claims for payment. Because the claims process does not require the documentation or maintenance of extraneous data, the data are thrown away.

First let's look at what documentation is kept and what data aren't kept. The patient demographics are kept for claims processing purposes, and these could be more valuable than in their current use (see below). The incidents of care consumption are recorded (e.g., diagnostic examinations and procedures and therapeutic procedures), along with their companion billing codes, including current procedural terminology (CPT) codes, Resource-Based Relative Value Scale (RBRVS) codes, DRG codes for inpatient procedures, Diagnostic Statistical Manual codes (DSM-4) for behavioral health-related claims, and/or International Classification of Disease codes (ICD-9-CM). On the surface, one would assume that all of the incidents of care consumption would be filed on the claim, yet data are still thrown away. For example, some providers utilize expected reimbursement-type computer software to determine which billing codes yield the most net revenues, meaning some procedures might not be recorded on the claim. On the other side, items included in the patient's chart but not included on the patient's claim form are likewise lost. These items include orders for pharmaceuticals (including over-the-counter medication) obtained by the patient at a community pharmacy, orders for consumable supplies that could represent noncovered charges, orders for home healthcare that might involve a separate claim (which often cannot be easily linked back to a patient's "master record" residing in the gatekeeper's office), procedures that the patient may elect to pay in cash and therefore do not necessitate filing a claim (e.g., inoculations against venereal disease, plastic surgery, and HIV tests), and procedures for which the provider might choose not to submit a claim (e.g., family courtesies or professional discretion).

The troubling aspect of such documentation is the limited purpose for which it may be used. Let's look at the process of submitting claims to a payor. A patient comes into an IPA's neighborhood clinic on Monday complaining of abdominal pain. A five-minute examination reveals nothing abnormal and the patient is prescribed an over-the-counter antacid. The same patient comes into the IPA's downtown clinic during lunch hour on Wednesday complaining of abdominal pain. After a five-minute exam that includes a review of the patient's record, the physician finds that another physician prescribed an antacid. The patient is rein-structed about taking the antacid, and a specific brand-name antacid (also over-the-counter) is prescribed. The same patient comes back to the IPA's neighborhood clinic on Friday complaining, again, of abdominal pain. After a five-minute examination and a blood test, the physician deter-mines that the patient is pregnant and refers her to a plan OB/GYN.

Let's review what occurred in the above scenario. The three incidents of care consumption involved a brief examination, perhaps a test, and a pre-scription (on Friday, prenatal vitamins were prescribed). The three clinic vis-its represent three distinct claims that the respective physicians can submit for payment. But let's look a little deeper, not into the substance of each visit, but into the longitudinal implications. The first two incidents of care con-sumption involved returns to the provider within 48 hours with the same pre-senting complaint. The obvious implication is that what was done on Monday and Wednesday *didn't have successful outcomes*. Since the IPA shared the same computer system for claims (remember that the provider on Wednesday, in a different location, was able to review the chart—meaning that the patient records are electronic—and to determine what was pre-scribed), that same physician should have known to try a different approach than the one used within the previous 48 hours. The physician seeing the pa-tient on Friday finally recognized that the patient had two consecutive nega-tive outcomes and took a different approach, which yielded an obvious situa-tion with an equally obvious resolution—the patient was pregnant all along. What would have happened if the Monday and Wednesday visits resulted in treatments or drugs which might have complicated the pregnancy? The physician was successful because he or she looked beyond the entitlement to file a claim for a visit and searched out different explanations to the three consecutive care consumption incidents for the same presenting complaint.

Another important aspect of the need for initial documentation con-cerns Medicare Risk populations. I stated in Chapter Five that the capita-tion management of Medicare Risk should optimally fall within a Reverse Gatekeeping® approach rather than in a highly profitable (to the payor only) traditional gatekeeping approach that utilizes HCFA's aver-age adjusted per capita as a means of setting very high capitation rates to which rationing-based strategies would be applied. The documentational need has to do with selective reassignment by the enrollee.

According to HCFA's rules for FQHMOs that receive approval to offer a Medicare Risk product, the Medicare beneficiary has the right to request a reassignment of his or her gatekeeper during the first 30 days of initially choosing a gatekeeper. Thus, to the chosen provider, the practice has 30 days (and usually less) to make a good impression on the Medicare beneficiary in order to hold on to the capitation for that individual and his or her spouse (if applicable). During this period, the Medicare beneficiary and his or her friends are checking out the provider. I believe that providers who can motivate their patients to lead healthy and productive lives can differentiate themselves with Medicare Risk enrollees and create a successful word-of-mouth promotional challenge to their colleagues.

At the same time that the Medicare Risk enrollees are choosing the "right" gatekeeper during their 30-day window, another 30-day window comes into play for the provider. The provider, too, has the right to request a reassignment of Medicare beneficiaries who choose him or her. Yet the selection criterion is not a smile or words of encouragement; rather, the litmus test involves the quantity and quality of information to determine whether there are the right attitudes, a malleable self-image, and other behaviors that can assist the provider in embarking on the path to self-managed health status improvements. I'm not advocating that providers selectively disenroll Medicare Risk enrollees on the basis of health status at the time of initial election. Besides appearing discriminatory to the enrollee and his or her friends, I doubt whether there is enough substance in judging an individual's will to succeed without observing behavior, demeanor, and self-image, since I believe that these are the documentable aspects of individuals becoming more motivated to create and improve on healthy lifestyles and eventual self-management of health status. In either event, documentation is a must, and the 30-day window means that the process of documenting new enrollees is critical to the success of capitated providers. The sooner that initial documentation is collected, whether for Medicare Risk or other capitation products, the sooner the provider can move into key capitation management strategies and actions.

This looking beyond the obvious consumption-based strategies of the old paradigm is what Disease State Management® is all about, but with a much larger payback for effort expended. With DSM populations for whom providers—hopefully specialty providers—are capitated, much of their remaining lives involves a disease progression. The long-term costs involved in managing disease state populations are much more significant management challenges than cross-sectional approaches aimed at managing individual incidents of consumption. For these populations, more significant financial returns are realized by how successfully DSM enrollees, on an individualized basis, adapt to their chronic conditions, improve their health, and reduce their need to consume expensive healthcare commodities more often.

For this population, the overall strategy involves spending some money on the front end to reduce more expensive outlays on the back end. For example, consumptive services spent on Type II diabetics, such as visits with a dietician; private health club memberships (that are subsidized only to the extent that the individual uses the benefit at least twice each week) with counseling by a trainer; and regular, periodic blood work, can have benefits far in excess of consumption spent by the capitated provider. In this example, the members of this DSM population can be taught how to reduce fat and increase fiber in their diet to effect healthy weight loss that can be sustained and, at the same time, eliminate the need for insulin and, perhaps, oral hypoglycemics; how to engage in appropriate exercise on a regular basis that sustains aerobic activity at a level that represents 85 percent of their target pulse rate, all aimed at aiding in healthy weight loss and in replacing fat tissue with muscle tissue which will reduce the tendency to return to obesity; and they will learn how to make adjustments in their lifestyle and eating habits to compensate for blood sugar fluctuations and maybe, just maybe, "cure" themselves of non-insulin-dependent diabetes mellitus—there is medical documentation that complete changes of lifestyle can bring about "remission." Variations of this strategy can also be applied to patients with hypertension, certain forms of cancer, coronary artery disease, previous congestive heart failure, chronic obstructive pulmonary disease, digestive disease (e.g., ulcerative colitis), and many others.

The items that need to be documented in the above example of diabetes involve more than the visits the patient has and the consumption on the part of the provider for which he or she may not be immediately reimbursed. The missing element is the enrollee's behavior. Provider observations of enrollees' behavior need to be documented and tracked within the electronic patient record. Inherent behaviors of individual enrollees, at the time they are initially screened (whether in a physician's office or at a gatekeeper open house, as described in Chapter Five) or at the time they enter into, or are assessed in conjunction with, a lifestyle improvement contract (see below), must be part of the record because it is behavior that is the longitudinal measurement used to determine if individuals are taking responsibility for their own health status.

In this case, the data most important for documentation are not the weight measurements, the interpretations of the radiologist in reading a smoker's chest X ray, or the lab results of a toxicology screen. No, the more important data are not for what you can bill but for what influences future consumptive activity: What is the patient's observed reaction to good news? Is he or she happy at the achievement or concerned that the results weren't good enough? Does the patient smile when the data indicate a less-than-optimal or even poor result? Does the patient seem depressed and beaten, or does he or she pledge to do better? More important to others who may be reviewing this scenario years later, how does the provider respond to a poorly motivated patient? Does the provider try to get the patient to recognize the bigger picture: that lasting, overall improvement in health status takes time, that one can't often turn around an entire life's progression over the course of a few months? Does the provider demonstrate to the patient that all efforts in the right direction are meritorious in and of themselves, and not just the biggest or most drastic incidents of improvement? Is the provider solicitous or genuine in his or her respect for the enrollee's efforts toward lifestyle improvement? What behaviors are occurring from both sides? All behaviors, positive and negative, should be observed. Videotaping behaviors could be advantageous, if the patient consents, in documentation, especially if the videotapes could be digitized and included within a multimedia electronic patient record system.

The demonstrated behavior to change is the catalyst that can lead to lasting effects on the overall progression of the disease state; the lifestyle change and the greater health status responsibility is the commodity that generates the payback for the provider and payor. For a Reverse Gatekeeper® provider, lifestyle improvement and documented behavior in assuming health status responsibility represents his or her return on investment (ROI).

Using Behavior Modification to Encourage Success

The onus for moving to the ROI behavior described above rests on the capitated enrollee, not on the provider. Hence, the first step is letting the enrollee know that his or her own behavior is important to the patient–provider relationship. One way this documentation can be done is if the enrollee is aware that a lifestyle improvement contract can be negotiated between the patient and the physician. Such a contract would be part of the patient's computerized profile that would be shared with other providers with whom the patient might seek care. The contract would involve the setting of lifestyle improvement objectives with scheduled assessment intervals, agreed to by both patient and provider. The progress in meeting such objectives can be reinforced by all providers who have authorized access to the patient's profile (e.g., members of the same IPA or group, contracted specialists who receive Reverse Gatekeeping® capitation, or members of the urgent care center or hospital emergency department that is provided institutional capitation in conjunction with the medical providers), so that they are part of a continuum of capitation management.

A strategy for enticing patients to consent to such a contract could involve offering incentives for meeting lifestyle improvement objectives or making measurable progress toward meeting each objective. Examples of such incentives could be monetary (e.g., $20 per pound of weight lost, $1,000 per year for avoiding obesity, $5 per pound of lost weight that is not regained), motivational (magazine subscriptions to a self-help publication, membership dues in a support organization, sponsorship in a walkathon, a charitable contribution to a medical research foundation, etc.), and/or personal (a smile, a kind word, and/or a demonstration of admiration or respect). People are best motivated if their actions please others, and doubly so if, in the process, they are pleasing themselves. The cost of offering incentives to others to achieve milestones in their personal lives is negligible compared with the rewards of a healthier lifestyle and a new outlook on beating their disease and/or minimizing the effects of the disease on leading a useful, productive life. Good health and healthy lifestyles should be associated with pleasure; this association is part of the behavior modification approach to wellness.

Feedback Loops

A principle of continuous quality improvement, especially when it entails introducing a change, involves collecting and managing feedback. The process by which evaluative information is collected and the results of all such collections shared with the respondents themselves is what is known as a *feedback loop*. In capitation management, the feedback loop defines and refines the relationship between the provider and the DSM patient or capitated enrollee, especially in measuring individuals' demonstrative progress in improving their lifestyle and in taking responsibility for their own health status.

As discussed previously, a provider's positive feedback for a job well done, evidenced both tangibly (with a cash or in-kind incentive) and intangibly (with words, gestures, and other nonverbal feedback), is a powerful motivator for change. In conjunction with both documentation and the above-referenced behavior modification, modeling approaches need to be taken under capitation management to assess whether incentives provided by the provider are being translated into demonstrable improvements in behavior related to lifestyle improvements and self-management of health status. This modeling approach, and the data generated (both documented gut feelings and actual test and observational results) represent the level of feedback that the provider should be generating for himself or herself for each capitated enrollee, especially so under a DSM approach. The level of sustained and measurable positive feedback the provider gives to the enrollee constitutes their feedback from the provider. The observable and documented reaction by the enrollee to the positive feedback generated by the provider to the enrollee is the basis of the provider's feedback from the enrollee. Yet even with both elements of feedback, there is no single feedback loop without relying on the scientific process.

The feedback loop is connected in the critical assessment of the appropriateness and success of feedback generated by both parties. The documentation of this assessment involves statistical modeling as part of enrollee wellness management or Disease State Management® services under capitation management. The responsibility of feedback documentation, because it forms the basis of documenting whether the goals of capitation management are achieved, should be considered too critical for a provider to delegate to others. Yet the ability to generate accurate feedback data and documentation, as well as reliable modeling approaches and the statistical reporting from such approaches, requires tremendous infrastructure. When capitation management is a more widespread activity, I envision that many MCOs will self-manage this critical process for feedback looping and may create a consulting arm that will contract with smaller providers and PSOs, probably on a subcapitated basis, to provide the documentation needed for evaluating capitation management success. I fully expect that a cottage industry will develop to manage the feedback loop and modeling applications, as well as suggest strategies for providing incentives that work better than others in influencing positive changes in enrollees' lifestyles and demonstrable improvements toward self-management of health status.

A final note on capitation management is in order. Much of this chapter describes a level of effort that does not yet exist. For most providers, capitation management remains a cost- and resource-management (minimization) approach or a piece of software, like EZ-CAP®, which providers utilize for managing capitation-related expenses, paying capitation vendors, adjusting staffing requirements, and rationing healthcare consumption resources. As a result, the concept of capitation management is just another extension to the insurance industry practice of redlining. The wellness and Disease State Management® aspects of capitation management are only now starting to emerge. I expect that we'll see a popularity of this aspect of capitation management among physicians involved in Reverse Gatekeeping.® I also expect that more of the health management side of capitation management will be occurring within currently immature or slowly maturing capitation markets. This expectation is not to say that mature capitation markets like Southern California will not experience wellness and Disease State Management® in what is now called capitation management. I expect that true capitation management will begin emerging among certain disease state populations capitated as part of a Reverse Gatekeeping® model in mature capitation markets like Southern California quite soon.

Chapter Seven

Capitation Opportunities for Vendors to Maximize

Vendors with whom I've talked over the last few years profess to know very little about managed care and capitation. I've found that they are in very good company. They have, by and large, never heard of the term *capitation*. Some jokingly reason that the term capitation has something to do with a French form of capital punishment. I often joke back that, under current market practices, a tie-in between capitation and decapitation isn't too far from the truth. Nevertheless, most have heard the term *managed care* yet again know very little about it other than what they read in the newspapers. With such a library, it's no wonder that capitated managed care is so poorly understood outside—and inside—the healthcare industry. In fact, most people who are truly aware of managed care perceive that it is a means by which physicians, hospitals, and the insurance industry will fight it out for whatever business remains. What few vendors truly realize is that the greatest market opportunities related to capitated managed care will be occurring *outside* the healthcare industry, not within it.

THE NEED FOR VENDOR CAPITATION

Let me show you where I'm heading with this analysis by providing two seemingly unrelated statistics. First of all, a growing number of medical economists, both inside and outside the private sector, are now predicting that between 50 and 80 percent of the healthcare industry will be capitated by the year 2000. In fact, some MCOs in Southern California are predicting nearly 80 percent capitation by the year 1998. Second, we know from government statistics that healthcare represents some 40 percent of the gross national product of the United States; yet only a portion of that 40 percent represents the billing activities of physicians and hospitals, not to mention premium sales of the health insurance industry. There is a tremendous amount of health-related business that occurs *outside* the healthcare and health insurance industries.

From my research, I've determined that there are many industries dependent on the healthcare industry for 50 percent or more of their sales. These industries include pharmaceutical companies, Baby Bell and regional telecommunications firms, medical instrumentation distributors, home medical equipment distributors, laboratory and radiological equipment manufacturers, manufacturers of sterile consumable supplies, manufacturers of sterilizing equipment, UNIX®-based computer manufacturers, distributors of janitorial supplies and chemical solvents, and biomedical waste disposal firms. These firms have defined sales objectives from business units within the healthcare industry that include hospitals, clinics, MCOs, physician offices, as well as ambulatory surgery and/or urgent care centers.

I often get these vendors to consider the issues related to capitated managed care when I inform them about the medical economists' predictions about future increases in capitation penetration, and followed up with a simple question: What are you doing *now* to protect the 50 percent or more of your business that will involve selling your goods and services to a capitated marketplace? Follow-up questions, for those who don't yet get it, include: When will you be up to speed on capitated managed care so that you can price your goods and services to allow your largest customers to still be able to buy from you after they become fully capitated? What will you do differently to price to, and service, capitated providers (who now represent over 50 percent of your business)? What changes to your charging and sales support infrastructures must you make within the next 2 1/2 to 5 years so that you'll be ready for substantial sales to capitated customers? How do you intend to position your goods and services and compete with similar vendors when the healthcare market is fully capitated?

VENDOR CAPITATION EFFECT ON STRENGTHENING CUSTOMER RELATIONSHIPS

As discussed in Chapter Six, providers who are capitated for 75 percent or more of their business will begin changing their costing and budgeting systems to reflect a PMPM reality. Yet how do vendors sell now? They sell on the basis of consumption and do not yet go at-risk according to levels of consumption; in fact, very few vendors are willing to accept consignment sales, which puts them even at negligible risk (e.g., for the speed of delivering such inventory). Pricing breaks are afforded on the basis of levels of consumption and vendors price their goods and services to be competitive or differentiated from their competitors who sell similar products for similar levels of consumption. Vendors charge their goods and services according to the consumption habits of their customers. Hence, their sales and selling strategies to healthcare customers presume that their consumption of such goods and services is entirely variable.

Yet it is exactly a turn away from variable costs and consumption on which capitated managed care is based! To providers who have reformulated their costing structures to a fixed, PMPM basis, variable consumption itself is a meaningless term. To the capitated group, all of their revenues are fixed (PMPM based) and great efforts are being undertaken to get their costs fixed as well. For budgeting purposes, the PMPM equivalent of each line item expense is used (e.g., equivalent purchased services per member per month, or dues and subscription expenses per member per month) rather than their consumptive-based values. Hence, expenses are identified according to their dollar impact on aggregate PMPM revenues.

The obvious question is therefore: How are vendors selling their products in ways that are convenient for the customer to purchase? A percentage discount off of total purchases made by the customer last year, assuming similar consumption levels, would have been highly desirable in a noncapitated environment but is meaningless in a capitated one. What is meaningful for the provider is to what extent vendors will go at-risk for reasonable levels of consumption and price their services on a PMPM basis.

VENDOR CAPITATION—PRICING STRATEGIES

Vendor pricing on a PMPM basis is not too difficult to conceptualize. Say a vendor budgets that it will generate $1 million in annual sales to a key healthcare client. Let's also say that the vendor needs to generate the same $1 million in sales each year for at least the next three years. The client MCO tells anyone who will listen that it has capitated responsiblities for 100,000 covered lives. How does the vendor approach pricing? The vendor would have to have a managed care products division to gather data on how its key customer consumes products purchased, in order to determine both what constitutes reasonable consumption levels, as well as the customer's history in over- and underconsumption. This division would provide specialized servicing to its managed care accounts (see below). In this process, the vendor would determine what net income it expects to generate from this MCO under a managed care pricing basis, divide the net income by 12 to derive a monthly net income, and then divide by the number of current covered lives to derive a PMPM price. Such pricing is typically offered on a three-year, exclusive basis at a given corridor of consumption (e.g., the reasonable consumption level plus or minus 10 percent over- or underusage). Consumption above the corridor would be paid by the MCO on the basis of a mutually agreeable price list; consumption below the corridor would be rebated by the vendor on the same price list basis.

VENDOR CAPITATION—COSTING STRATEGIES

In terms of deriving net income, the vendor must carefully analyze the quantity and quality of its truly fixed and variable costs for a capitated customer. In this regard, the vendor's finance department must pay particular attention to deductions from revenue (e.g., subcapitation fees paid by providers, which are the very first to be paid); truly fixed expenses (e.g., the necessity of the same levels of sales and customer relations staff for a capitated customer's guaranteed volume of business); variable expenses (e.g., whether detailers have to expend the same level of effort for customers with relatively fixed volume); and incremental expenses (e.g., customer consumption-related modeling studies). This approach needs to be taken for each customer to whom capitated pricing will be offered. Given the uniqueness of this level of effort, creating a separate managed care division to generate these analyses leading to PMPM pricing would be advised. A separate division is also advisable given the differences in the way the vendor will choose to manage capitated accounts.

The biggest difference in the way the vendor will service the account has to do with the concept of bearing risk. Currently, vendors bear little, if any, risk for the levels of services and products sold to their customers. In a parallel manner, capitated customers increasingly perceive that they need to cut their costs, especially as they relate to the providers' overhead. As a result, they are cutting back on their consumption of services, which is serving to jeopardize the vendors' sales expectations. Where customers aren't cutting back, many vendors feel that they need to provide differentiated service (zero-defect products, more detailers visiting the customer more often, heightened customer service and convenience, etc.) to fulfill new and retained sales objectives. In another result, the healthcare customers are setting restrictions on the way the vendor does his or her job, motivated solely on the basis of cost savings (e.g., developing formularies for pharmaceutical products, accepting shipments only on specified days, specifying which days vendor sales staff can be present in the hospital). Most infuriating of all for vendors is the typical increase in the Days in Accounts Payable for many vendors (from 90 to 180 days in accounts payable is not uncommon), which is leading to both increases in bad-debt expenses as well as increased collections expenses.

VENDOR CAPITATION POSITIONING OBJECTIVES

A real bonus for vendors caught in these cost-cutting moves by healthcare customers is that capitated pricing frees vendors to develop their own process for servicing the customer most efficiently. Since the risk has already been capitated, a vendor can set up its own best practices in servicing the account. Capitated pharmaceutical firms might feel that they can better guarantee the quality of their merchandise to the customer if patients receive name-brand drugs instead of generics. Instrumentation firms may wish to supply the customer entirely on a consignment basis. A minor consumables supplier subject to capitated pricing may choose to have detailers on the customer's premises every morning to ensure that a guaranteed supply of product is available on a continuous basis.

In short, those who bear the risk are no longer micromanaged in terms of how they choose to manage that risk. If a vendor is capitated to manage a hospital's materials management function on an outsourced basis, it might choose to upgrade to bar-coding—at the vendor's sole expense— to achieve greater supply cost savings than it would have been able to guarantee without the benefit of modern technology. Vendors will naturally choose the most cost-effective means of delivering consistent supply at consistent quality. Furthermore, such vendors are much more qualified to manage their own business than most any customer will ever be.

OTHER FORMS OF VENDOR CAPITATION

So far, I've discussed the most obvious type of vendor and the most obvious type of vendor motivation in looking toward a capitated marketplace in the healthcare industry. Let's also consider other partnering relationships. I mentioned in Chapter Six about the needs for longitudinal health profiles and modeling approaches regarding feedback loops between providers and their capitated enrollees, particularly within DSM populations. Nothing presumes that providers, and even the largest MCOs, will have the wherewithal to self-manage these functions. Yet vendors can generate a win–win approach by partnering with their healthcare customers, particularly their capitated ones, in co-developing these processes and/or in tracking data that could lead to an ambulatory outcomes data set. For example, one of the critical commodities in performing these modeling studies is a large computer with ample storage and report-writing capabilities. A key vendor with this capability is a healthcare collections agency. Therefore, in this example, perhaps a healthcare collections agency, if approached, may wish to partner with an MCO for purposes of performing modeling studies on behalf of the MCO's providers and capitated enrollees, all for a capitated price or a quid pro quo for noncapitated business.

Another vendor positioning strategy is truly outside the realm of the old paradigm. In a capitated world, a capitated medical group would love to be able to pay a single check to a vendor consortium that would provide all nonmedical services for a single capitated price. Thus, a new form of MSO could be created in that the organization would enter into capitated pricing with a full spectrum of vendors with whom medical providers might desire to contract. The MSO would charge an administrative add-on fee to the total of capitated pricing negotiated with all of the vendors. The MSO would then fix a single PMPM price that the provider pays this consortium; the MSO, in turn, then pays each of the vendors its capitated fee, and the vendors bear the capitated risk—and provide customer services—directly with the purchasing provider organization.

I don't believe that any measurable progress is being made in this area of consortium-based vendor capitation because of lack of insight, as well as the fact that the types of vendors with whom capitated providers now contract are quite diverse. They are so diverse, in fact, that there is an absence of networking among the different vendors. For example, how often does a janitorial supply firm have a need to talk with a home health agency or a radiographic film supplier? How rare is it that any of these three vendors would ever find themselves in the same room together, let alone on the same side of a bargaining table? The real opportunity is in switching the paradigm and looking "outside the box."

Epilogue

A Vision for the Future

So much of this book has seemed so obvious to me for so many years now that I am dumbfounded that so little has really been written on the nonfinancial rationale for capitation, the strategies that make capitation successful in today's marketplace as well as in emerging capitation markets, and the strategies that vendors should be taking in repositioning their businesses for a capitated healthcare marketplace. In short, I can't understand why such a book has not yet been written. I consider myself fortunate to have fulfilled a life's dream to commit my often renegade views about capitation to paper and to have received the guidance and support of Irwin Professional Publishing toward this end.

I'd like to take this final opportunity to look into the future, especially as it relates to capitated managed care. My greatest vision is that the Reverse Gatekeeping® approach trademarked by CompCare will form the basis for an entirely new managed care system that would operate in a parallel manner to traditional gatekeeping. Reverse Gatekeeping® represents a managed care strategy that can create a new lifeblood for America's hospitals, especially its teaching hospitals, and can enhance the businesses and skill levels of our specialists who, in mature capitation markets, have experienced severe cutbacks in patient volumes and have in some cases been forced into bankruptcy. I am so confident of the value of Reverse Gatekeeping®, especially in its applicability to Medicare Risk populations, that I feel this new system can resurrect the Medicare and Medicaid programs, instill a new faith by Americans in the managed care concept, and bring back a doctor–patient relationship to the 1990s that few people would ever associate with HMOs, public health, and managed care.

I believe that people want to improve their health, take stock of their lifestyles, and begin to take more responsibility for their health status. I feel that providers who respect and admire the efforts of their DSM population to improve their own health, and who offer incentives to them accordingly, will be the ones most successful at achieving excellent long-term outcomes, successful adaptations to disease states, and enhanced wellness. Capitated enrollees will respect their providers more if they are allowed to manage their own lives with the guidance, counsel, respect, admiration, and acceptance of their providers. In the process, the providers improve their own reputation in the eyes of the communities they serve, and the payor's ability to sell premium is enhanced by the outcomes, reputation, and commitment to quality of its providers.

The obstacles toward achieving this vision for the future do not rest in what passes for managed care today, nor are they the fault of capitation. The real obstacles are of our own creation. They reflect our unwillingness to shift our paradigms and our unwillingness to challenge our assumptions concerning provider motivations in a capitated world and their relationships with other consumers and providers. **We can change the paradigm at any time.** We can find ways to make our efforts successful, rather than focusing on the obvious brass ring of short-term profit and rationing. I expect that time will show that providers who offer a differentiated capitation management product will experience far greater profitability and prestige than some of the dominant groups and IPAs that negotiate strictly on the basis of price.

With 80 percent of the market going to capitation within the next 10 years, and in all likelihood much sooner than that, capitated managed care truly represents our future. My vision of the future is that capitation will be much different than it is today, and will focus on both traditional and Reverse Gatekeeping® approaches, depending on the disease or wellness classification of any one enrollee. Capitation will represent financial rewards for those who truly understand it and maximize the opportunities inherent in a new health delivery construct. The success of these new opportunities depends on providers' willingness to change, to accept the new paradigm, and to rise to the challenge. It surely won't be long now.

About the Author

David I. Samuels, MPA, CMCP

Mr. Samuels is a nationally recognized authority on capitated managed care development and future directions. Mr. Samuels is currently vice president, Development for Comprehensive Care Corporation, charged with developing a diverse portfolio of capitation-based disease management products utilizing state-of-the-art computerized technologies. He is also a member of the faculty of the Health Sciences Department at Chapman University, teaching healthcare management, healthcare finance, and capitated managed care within its Masters of Healthcare Administration program. Mr. Samuels is a member of the program faculty within the Center of Excellence in Health Care Management at the University of Southern California, with teaching responsibilities in the areas of capitated managed care, clinical practice parameters, and development of clinical and service outcomes. As a consultant, Mr. Samuels has been educating the public sector to take advantage of private-sector opportunities in the field of capitated managed care. Mr. Samuels is an advanced member of the Healthcare Financial Management Association with professional distinction as a Certified Managed Care Professional; he has been a member of the Southern California Chapter's Board of Directors since 1991, is widely published within his chapter, and has received numerous local and national awards for both professional and personal service.

INDEX

Other books of interest to you from Irwin Professional Publishing . . .

THE FOR-PROFIT HEALTHCARE REVOLUTION
The Growing Impact of Investor-Owned Health Systems
Sandy Lutz and E. Preston Gee
ISBN: 1-55738-650-1

THRIVING ON REFORM
Meeting Tomorrow's Healthcare Challenges Today
E. Preston Gee
ISBN: 1-55738-618-8

NOT WHAT THE DOCTOR ORDERED
Reinventing Medical Care in America
Jeffrey C. Bauer
ISBN: 1-55738-620-X

STRATEGIC HEALTHCARE MANAGEMENT
Applying the Lessons of Today's Top Management Experts to the Business of Managed Care
Ira Studin
ISBN: 1-55738-631-5

HEALTHCARE MARKETING IN TRANSITION
Practical Answers to Pressing Questions
Terrence J. Rynne
ISBN: 1-55738-635-8